```
RC          Johnson, Edwin T.
280
.B8         Breast cancer, black
J64            woman.
1993


$19.75
```

	DATE		

CHICAGO PUBLIC LIBRARY
NORTH AUSTIN BRANCH
5724 W. NORTH AVE. 60639

BAKER & TAYLOR

BREAST CANCER BLACK WOMAN

EDWIN T JOHNSON, MD

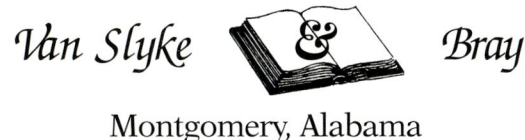

Van Slyke & Bray
Montgomery, Alabama

About The Cover

The art work on the cover comes from a greeting card, circa 1965—painter unknown. It depicts a youthful and an older black woman as they sit together, perhaps discussing the commonplace subjects of the day. The women are dressed with color and spark, and yet they remain reserved and demure. The lines of the older woman speak of age and sagacity acquired by living and surviving. The younger woman appears alert and fresh—attentive to the admonitions and guidance of her elder. These are the women who cradle our future. Both are vulnerable to breast cancer. They deserve, nay, command! our respect and protection.

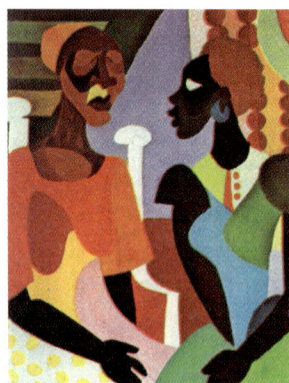

Copyright© 1993 by Van Slyke & Bray. All rights reserved. No part of this work may be reproduced or transmitted in any form or by any means, electronic or mechanical, including photocopying and recording, or by any information storage or retrieval system, except as may be expressly permitted by the 1976 Copyright Act or in writing from the publisher. Requests for permission should be addressed in writing to Van Slyke & Bray, 4152-C Carmichael Road, Montgomery, Alabama 36106.

Design, composition and film by Compos-It, Inc., Montgomery, Alabama.
The text is set in New Aster and Frutiger.

ISBN: 0-9635435-0-4   Library of Congress Catalog No. 92-062442   ©Copyright No. TXu 439-457

First Printing 12/93   Printed in the U.S.A.

Dedicated to

African American Women

and those who love them

TABLE OF CONTENTS

iii   PREFACE

v   INTRODUCTION

1   CHAPTER I

WHEN THE SHOE'S ON THE OTHER FOOT—
The Patient's Point of View (and my thoughts, too)

21   CHAPTER II

WHERE IT ALL BEGINS—
Breast Development, Construction and Function

35   CHAPTER III

A CASE FOR SHERLOCK HOLMES—
Making the Diagnosis

59   CHAPTER IV

THE FICKLE FINGER OF FATE—
Who Gets Breast Cancer?

87   CHAPTER V

A NEEDLE IN THE HAYSTACK—
Finding Breast Cancer

101   CHAPTER VI

NO NEWS IS GOOD NEWS—RIGHT? WRONG!
Know your Enemy to Survive

113   CHAPTER VII

THE BATTLE PLAN—
What is the Best Treatment for Breast Cancer Today?

141   CHAPTER VIII

LIGHTS, CAMERA, ACTION!
The Show Must Go On

The cast of characters involved in the national breast cancer debate has taken on a different hue. Dr Johnson has written a timely dissertation and added a new dimension to the breast cancer epidemic as it relates to the Black woman. Dr Johnson has given to us, Black women, the perspective we need to be able to continue to argue the issues of health care reform, breast cancer screening guidelines and the relationship between early detection and treatment and our survival.

Zora Kramer Brown, Founder and Chairperson Breast Cancer Resource Committee Washington, DC (14 year breast cancer survivor)

PREFACE

*e*very year more...women die from breast cancer because they do not receive mammograms and breast exams as often as they should. One out of every nine women will be diagnosed with breast cancer.... This year (1992) an estimated 46,000 women will die from breast cancer...1500 more than in 1991, and 180,000 new cases will be discovered.

But breast cancer is particularly devastating in our nation's black women. ...Breast cancer is currently the leading cause of cancer death for African-American women. The National Cancer Institute estimates that over 44,000 black women died from breast and cervical cancer in the last decade.

Only 58 percent of African American women 40 and older have ever received a mammogram. Within the next decade, the lives of more than 13,000 black women could be saved by simply getting regular mammograms and clinical breast examinations.

...when detected early...breast cancer can be treated with radiation or chemotherapy which can reduce the need for radical surgery....90 percent of women who are diagnosed early...will survive breast cancer...

...too many women think it won't happen to them and delay regular clinical breast examinations and mammograms until it is too late....

Learn and practice monthly self-breast examination.... The cost of breast cancer screenings are between $50 and $150.

...there are ...organizations..and other agencies that have low-cost or free mammography services....

If you have never had a breast exam, don't put it off any longer. Early breast cancer detection can be a choice between life and death. For your sake choose prevention and early detection. Choose life.

Louis W Sullivan, MD
former Secretary of Health and Human Services

condensed from an article (BREAST CANCER IN BLACK WOMEN)

INTRODUCTION

Several years ago I had the occasion to participate in a 'health education fair' sponsored by one of those missionary circles that are found in every black Baptist church. I could have chosen to speak on hypertension or sickle-cell anemia, both important topics in the black community. But I had recently operated on a twenty-six year old black woman with breast cancer, and I decided this was an opportunity to remind these church women of the danger signals of breast cancer and the importance of early detection.

As I began to review the literature in preparation for my talk, I was surprised to learn that black women, young and old, were contracting breast cancer at an ever alarming rate, especially in the 30 to 50 year old age group. At the same time I found that the incidence was stabilizing among whites.

I also discovered that more black women with breast cancer had a spreading malignancy when first discovered; and fewer white women had advanced breast cancer when first seen. So the cure rate for black women was lower. Even when breast cancer was detected at a comparable stage, the chance for survival, for obscure reasons, was much worse among black women. And finally, I found that black women were caught up in myth and mis-information regarding cancer in general and breast cancer in particular.

Obviously, I had to conclude: **Black women are at special risk.** So instead of just a general review of the danger signals of breast cancer, I felt this 'health education fair' was a perfect opportunity to give these black women information that pertained to them directly. As far as I could observe there was little concerted effort on the global scene to warn the black community of their peculiar vulnerability to breast cancer.

Certainly current resources available to the community were inadequate to address many of the common health issues facing black people, much less focus on breast cancer. But individual effort might make a difference. If speaking to small groups such as this health fair had merit, then addressing a wider audience should have an even greater impact. Perhaps a book directed towards black women and their families was part of the solution.

I reviewed the medical literature, and sought the opinion of leading authorities and colleagues. I talked to nurses and therapists. I interviewed cancer patients and their families; and pondered my own personal surgical experience in treating breast cancer, which was occasionally rewarding, but too often too late and tragic.

The idea of a book? Why not! A book that would alert black women and not frighten them, would counsel and not preach. A book that would inform and challenge. A book with a title that was not fancy but would get right to the matter. Aha! But how to go from an idea into reality—from blank sheet to something tangible?

There were no short cuts. It was a process of distilling the information, rewriting, reworking, rethinking, rechecking, updating, and repeating the process again and again. Eventually my thoughts were shaped and crystallized into this volume: BREAST CANCER/ BLACK WOMAN.

Chapter one is a fictional discussion, based on a composite of factual interviews with real breast cancer patients. Chapter Two is a molding of several past group presentations, designed to emphasize the anatomical basis for breast cancer. In Chapter Three through Eight aspects of breast cancer are examined through various approaches for clarity and understanding.

The drawings on the rear cover of the book and in Chapters Two and Three are used with the permission of Techpool, Inc, Romaine Pierson Publishers, Inc, and J B Lippincott Company.

My thanks to Dr Claude Organ, Professor of Surgery, who took the time to encourage my efforts. I am also indebted to Dr George Crile Jr, and Dr Bernard Fisher for their wisdom and support along the way.

I am grateful to the women who were kind enough to relate to me their personal experiences that gave me insight and provided the catalyst to complete this work.

And thank you to Helen Shambray-Johnson for constructive criticism and for copy-editing the manuscript.

―――

The goals of BREAST CANCER/BLACK WOMAN are threefold:

The first goal is to cut through the maze of misinformation and make the reader aware that breast cancer can be cured when discovered early.

The second goal is to emphasize that every woman should play a vital integral part in detecting breast cancer at an early favorable stage.

The third goal is to encourage black women to evaluate the options now available in the care of breast cancer and participate in treatment decisions.

Knowledge can be life-saving
My people are destroyed for lack of knowledge—Hosea 4:6

CHAPTER ONE

WHEN THE SHOE'S ON THE OTHER FOOT
The Patient's Point of View (and my thoughts, too)

*P*hysicians and care givers must continually ask themselves the question, 'How would I respond if I were the patient? How would I want to be treated? What if the shoe was on the other foot?'

That question has been constantly before me as a physician whenever I've been called upon to give an injection, or pass a tube, or repair a laceration or in some way to inflict discomfort.

When a particular procedure promises to be uncomfortable or downright painful, I tell the patient, 'I'm pretending I'm doing this to myself, so you know I'll be careful.' It's amazing how one can reduce the discomfort with that simple thought. It might mean waiting a few minutes to locate a smaller catheter, or using a smaller needle, or taking the time to numb the throat when passing a stomach tube. All sorts of things come to mind when you consciously put yourself in the patient's shoes.

Have you ever noticed bad it hurts when someone uses a pin to remove a splinter from your finger? But when you do it to yourself, it doesn't hurt nearly as much. That's because you automatically do whatever you can to avoid pain that you will feel while you

> *Before 1975, treatment options for breast cancer were not generally explained to the patient by most surgeons. Today a new era of doctor-patient relationship is upon us. Patients no longer need to accept whatever is offered, oblivious of other choices. It is no longer acceptable to let questions go unanswered.*

remove the splinter from your own finger. It's simply human nature.

I believe all care-givers should respond in human terms to that question, 'What if I were the patient and the shoe was on the other foot'. For surely as we live, the toll of time will eventually place all of us in that circumstance.

This chapter is for the care-givers—not only the medical professionals, but even more for the patients' loved ones—the husband and off-springs, the well-wishers, the friends, even the casual acquaintances. It's time for **all** of us to be caring givers, to appreciate the breast cancer dilemma through the experience of the patient. Hopefully this awareness will heighten our empathy and sensitivity and help us lend our support and understanding in finding a coping strategy.

Before 1975, treatment options for breast cancer were not generally explained to the patient by most surgeons; and, in those days that was perfectly permissible. When a patient was anesthetized, she understood that if the biopsy was positive for cancer, radical surgery was to be done before waking her. If the patient awoke without a breast, obviously there was cancer. And that was acceptable treatment. Few doctors asked the question, 'How would I want to be treated?'

Nowadays, however, in several states the doctor, by law, is required to make breast cancer patients aware of all available treatment options.[3] Medical information is now available to the public as never before. People are generally more informed, and often insist on making their own decisions, or at least be a part of the decision making process. The doctor today, to be in step with the times, must give his patient that option.

A new era of doctor-patient relationship is upon us. Patients no longer need to accept whatever is offered, oblivious of other choices. It is no longer acceptable to let questions go unanswered or simply to observe a breast lump because the doctor said so. The second most common medico-legal allegation filed against physicians is due to the failure to diagnose breast cancer.[2]

Women must be alert and doctors must be aggressive in uncovering breast cancer. This particularly is the case in black women under age 35 where breast cancer is one and a half times as frequent as in the white population[1]; and then the patient must be informed regarding available treatments and involved in the making of sometimes difficult choices.

Hopefully information in this book will provide women and their families a better understanding of breast cancer, particularly in the black community, and encourage them to openly discuss their needs and concerns with their health providers and to be an active participant in treatment decisions.

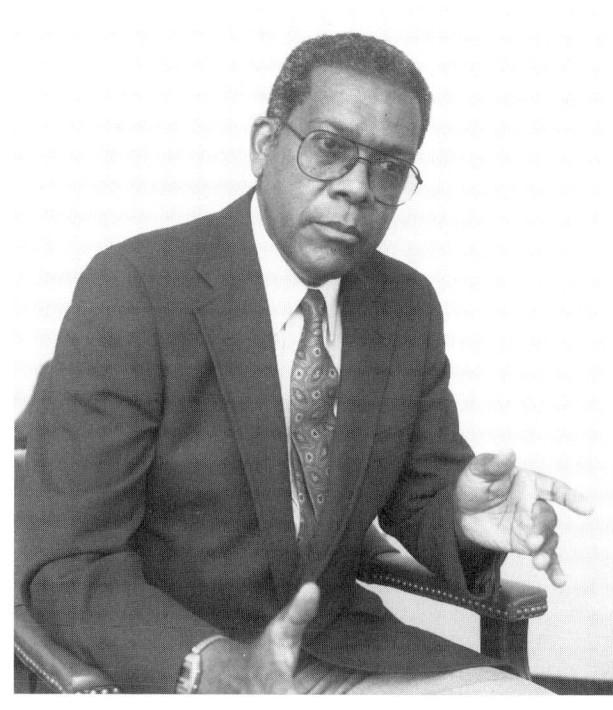

Women must be alert and doctors must be aggressive in uncovering breast cancer. This particularly is the case in black women under age 35 where breast cancer is one and a half times as frequent as in the white population.

I interviewed a number of black women who had been treated for breast cancer before 1975. None of them was my personal patient. I found them through oncology nurses, social workers, medical colleagues and simply word of mouth. I learned of their experiences with their doctors, the hospital staff, the reaction of their husbands and family, and their adjustment in the work place. I believed that the viewpoints

Peggy Thornton was a 37-year-old single parent. She discovered breast cancer, and then faced an emotional roller coaster of fear, disgust, divorce and finally accommodation.

• • • • • • •

of black women from different age groups and backgrounds who had actually lived through those trying days should be recorded and passed on to enhance our sensitivity and make all of us more understanding and aware of this cancer epidemic.

I reviewed my notes from numerous interviews and discovered that none of these women were given any real opportunity to participate in their treatment decisions; and several had stories of depression and misgiving. Others related insensitivity at the hands of medical people and lack of support from loved ones.

I decided to incorporate these viewpoints into three fictional women of diverse backgrounds and allow them to openly describe their impressions, and talk about how they coped with their cancer—to convey the psychological impact of breast cancer. Let me introduce these fictional characters as they relate their experiences:

1. Peggy Thornton was a 37-year-old single parent who had discovered breast cancer some time in 1968, had a mastectomy in 1970, and then faced an emotional roller coaster of fear, disgust, divorce and finally accommodation. She survived an ordeal and now, for several years has worked as a bank officer.

2. Mrs Foster, on the other hand, was in her late sixties, overweight, bent with arthritis, and on medication for high blood pressure. She'd been married for over 40 years and had raised a family before finding a knot in her breast and undergoing mastectomy about 1972.

3. Mrs Beatrice Robinson, a 52-year-old housewife who had had a mastectomy in 1974, had adjusted fairly well, and had good support from family and friends. She blamed her doctor for not finding her cancer sooner.

Let's pretend that these fictional characters gathered in my office at my invitation to talk about their experiences. I'll start the discussion:

"In a few days I'm scheduled to speak on breast cancer and the black family. I would like to relay some of the problems faced by patients with their doctors and with the hospital staff. Tell me about attitudes you faced at home and on the job. I want you to help me to understand what it's like when the shoe's on the other foot."

Peggy Thornton spoke up right away. "Well, I think it's high time somebody tried to find out what patients feel and how we do after the surgery's all over. I'll be happy to tell you how I got along. I had this white doctor. They're supposed to be so good, no offense, Dr Johnson; but that doctor didn't tell me a thing. He was just too cold and impersonal. I didn't even know he was going to remove my breast."

It would seem that Mrs Thornton was not pleased with her doctor. And this is the dilemma I've heard time and time again. Black women and their families naturally want the best medical care possible; and black folks, in general, actually believe the white man's ice is colder. We may be able to out-run, out-jump, out-rap and out-dance the white man, but when it comes to serious business, so many of us make haste to submit our treasure and our bodies to the man, having been taught in so many subtle ways that the white pilot, the white lawyer, or anything white has more innate knowledge and skill.

In the same vein, many black women opt for a surgeon who looks like Jesus and quickly overlook the doctor's cool detached attitude so long as the skin is white and the hair is flaxen. I recall patients who've sought a second opinion (code for preferring a white doctor), only to be put to sleep and then actually operated on by a doctor in training, while her surgeon looked over the trainee's shoulder or retreated to the lounge for a Coke or cigarette.

I also vividly remember being called as a friend of the family to give my opinion regarding a desperately ill patient with liver cancer at the VA Hospital in San Francisco. The patient had obviously expired. I examined my friend carefully. He was still hooked up to IV fluids and a mechanical breathing apparatus. The nurses had been waiting about 30 minutes for a doctor to come and pronounce the patient dead, and in the interim the family had called me at my office to come and, I thought, to give my opinion. I left an office full of patients to be at the side of this family in this crisis; and I tried to explain as tenderly as possible that this good husband

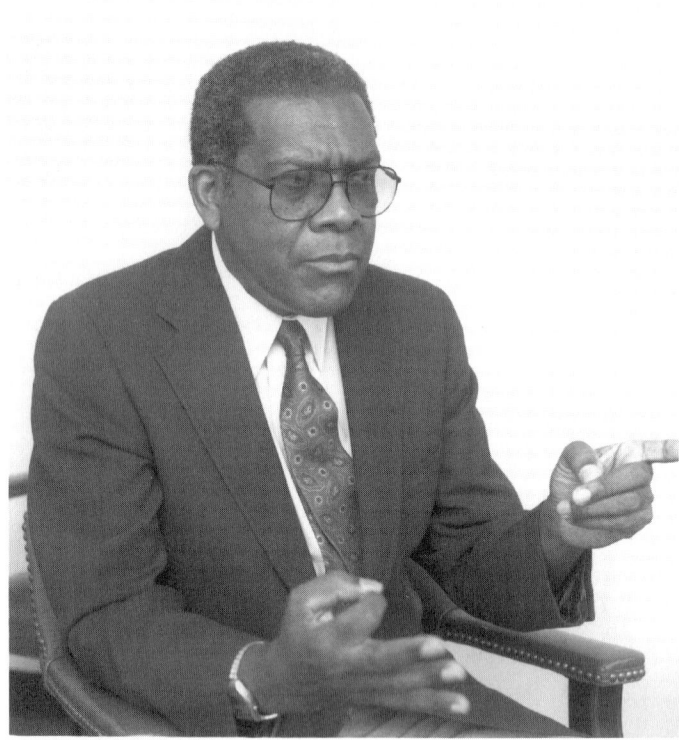

We may be able to out-run, out-jump, out-rap and out-dance the white man, but when it comes to serious business, so many of us have been taught in so many subtle ways that the white pilot, the white lawyer, or anything white has more innate knowledge and skill.

and father was gone. No one said a word. There was no emotion. The drip of the IV continued. The grind of the respirator and the rhythmic heave of the thorax proceeded. I suspected the wife was in shock, so I whispered again to the deceased's brother, "I believe he's gone, Robert."

"We're waiting for the doctor", replied Robert. After another fifteen minutes or so, watching the chest go up and down, Dr Jesus breezed in followed by two nurses holding medical charts. He took one look, waved his stethoscope across the chest, turned to the

> *I'd been going to my doctor for diabetes but he never checked my breast. I had to find it myself. I was just lying on the couch watching television. I guess I was scratching or rubbing my breast when I felt this knot.*
> ● ● ● ● ● ●

nurses and exclaimed to the group, "This man is dead." He looked at the nurses, "Remove the respirator and IV's." And then he was gone, no personal words to the family. Nothing.

In an instant the seven or eight family members around the bed let up a holler. You talk about wailing and gnashing of teeth. They hugged each other, screamed and sobbed. In the melee someone thanked me for coming. And I slipped away feeling my ice was not quite as cold as I thought it was.

Therefore I understood very well where Peggy was coming from. Black physicians immersed in the quagmire of medical racism on a daily basis, must also tolerate a cool aloofness from white colleagues. But this was not a time to voice my own opinion or experiences. This discussion was about learning from these women—how they coped and responded to **their** own personal experiences. So I proceeded.

"Alright ladies lets begin by throwing out a question for you. "How did you happen to discover the lump in your breast. Was it your own finding or did a doctor or nurse find it on routine examination."

Mrs Robinson, who had a mastectomy in 1974, began to speak. "I'd been going to my doctor for diabetes but he never checked my breast. I had to find it myself. I was just lying on the couch watching television. I guess I was scratching or rubbing my breast when I felt this knot.

Again, I sensed that the doctor or the system was being blamed. "How long had you been going to that doctor for diabetes, Mrs Robinson?"

"Oh, for years." "And he never gave you a complete examination?" "He probably did a long time ago, but nothing regularly. He would just check my sugar and write prescriptions."

"Okay, tell us about this knot you found." "I didn't think too much of it at the time. But I noticed it a few days later while in the bathtub. I told my husband and he thought I should have it checked. I knew it couldn't be a cancer because it didn't hurt or nothing. Then I kind of forgot all about it until I noticed it was growing."

"And how long did that take." "I guess it was about six months later." "Did you tell your doctor then?" "No I didn't. I kind of thought it might be an infection or something. I guess I was hoping it **wasn't** a cancer. I was hoping it would go away. But then my arm started swelling and I finally told my doctor. He referred me for surgery right away."

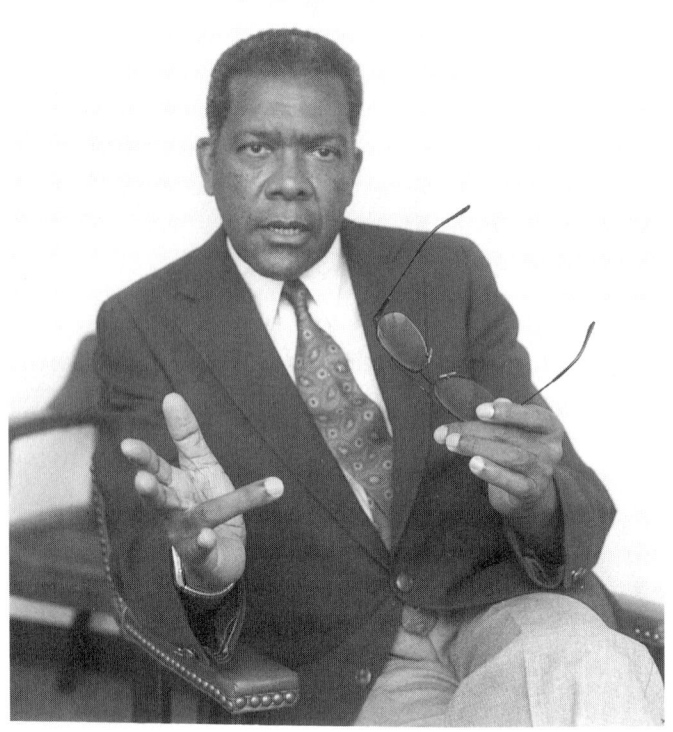

Did any of your doctors sit down and explain other choices of treatment?

"How much time passed between the time you first noticed the lump and finally had surgery?"

"It must have been over a year, Doctor Johnson." "But you saw your doctor for diabetes and probably other things during that time!"

"Yes, but be didn't check my breast and I guess I didn't tell him about it. Don't ask me why. I know I should have", she smiled.

I suppose it's easier to blame the system, I thought. But shouldn't the patient take some responsibility also?

"You had the breast removed, I understand. Were you given any other treatment choices?"

"No, the surgeon said that this was the best way to

go and I thought that he, being the doctor, knew best. I never even thought to question anything."

"What about you, Peggy? What were the circumstances when you first noticed something was wrong?"

Peggy Thornton had gone on to complete her degree in business administration since her mastectomy in 1970. She was now in the management training program at one of the leading banks. She was a divorcee and was raising a teenage daughter with the help of her mother, who lived with her.

"I first was aware that a lump was in my breast when I accidentally bumped myself on a sack of groceries I was holding and leaning on, trying to get my key in the front door. It hurt a little and at first I thought I bruised my breast, but later I checked and found this knot. It didn't feel like a bruise and I immediately thought of cancer. But would you believe I was too scared to see a doctor or even to talk about it.

When I did go to this black doctor, his receptionist asked me right out in front of everyone in the waiting room what my problem was. She was behind a counter but still everybody in the room could hear. I told her I wanted to speak to the doctor privately and she tells me that I had to tell her first. You know how we are when we get a little job. I could have kicked her behind right there, but I was cool. I told her I'd return later but I was so embarrassed I never went back.

"For about a year I kept putting it off and hoping the lump would go away. It didn't seem to be getting any bigger and I guess I really hoped it would eventually go away. Then I got this lump under my armpit, and that's when I mentioned it to my husband."

"How did he respond?" "Horrible. He was in the middle of working on his Masters degree and trying

I first was aware that a lump was in my breast when I accidentally bumped myself on a sack of groceries I was holding and leaning on, trying to get my key in the front door. For about a year I kept putting it off and hoping the lump would go away.

• • • • • • •

to hold down a job. Our daughter was only ten and I guess the pressure was too much for him. He just balled me out for not telling him sooner. He just couldn't or wouldn't understand how scared I was even though I knew it was probably a cancer. We weren't getting along too good anyway but we started having more fights. He didn't want to even get close to me. Then my sister told me about this white doctor at the medical center. He was supposed to be a good surgeon and all that. But, Lord knows, he was so cold—I mean chilly!—if you know what I mean (I did). I don't think he ever looked me in the eye once. He said he'd do a biopsy and remove the breast if it was a cancer; but he wasn't sure it was a cancer and not to worry about it. So I didn't really think they were going to cut off my breast even though I signed a consent form. To me that consent form meant: 'I trust you to do the right thing'.

"After surgery I woke up with this huge bandage on my chest. I wasn't hurting much at first, but I was scared. I was so depressed and angry, but what could I do? My husband was acting like a robot. We hardly even spoke when he came to the hospital. I was a mess. My chest looked so bad when they changed the dressing I cried. It was terrible. I had no idea it would look so bad, and the doctor talking about how good it was healing. A radical mastectomy. Can you imagine?

"My little girl wanted to know what was happening. My husband was withdrawn, and my momma talkin' about 'give it time'. My arm started swelling and my shoulder got stiff. The surgeon seemed too busy to give me much time. Even the interns, you know, the student doctors seemed too busy to talk much.

"When I finally got home I couldn't find the right kind of bra for weeks. Clothes wouldn't fit right. I got my hair done—it didn't look right. Her eyes rolled up and a sigh whistled through her teeth. "I tell you, for a while it was pure hell."

"Well, we can be thankful you've managed to come this far, Peggy. You've been fortunate to have no residual arm swelling or shoulder stiffness. I think you've shown you've got what it takes to overcome. Now, what about you, Mrs Foster? We haven't heard from you. Tell us how you discovered you had a breast cancer." Did you get the support you thought you needed at home?

Mrs Foster, plump and gray in a flowered house dress, was almost seventy years old. She seemed content and adjusted in spite of the chronic swelling of her right arm, held in check by an elastic sleeve. She gave us a broad smile.

"Well, you see, Doctor Johnson, I been married about 45 years and me and Jim, my husband, we'd seen a lots together, children all grown and everything. My husband had that prostrate surgery a few years before my surgery, so he couldn't do much in the way of sex anyways, so our relationship didn't really change that much."

I hadn't asked about sex relations, but this simply pointed out that regardless of age, sex is not far from the topic of conversation even at age sixty-nine.

"In fact he was real nice to me when I was sick", said Mrs Foster. "I guess I wasn't looking for him to be mean or nothing. Truth is he's always been good to me. And my children still come around reg'lar—makes it nice. Even when they brings theys children for me to mind."

She smiled broadly again and the rest of us responded. "Tell us how you found out there was something wrong with your breast?"

"I was dressing—putting on my clothes, when I felt this hard knot in my breast. 'Bout the size of the end of my finger. It didn't hurt or nothin'. (Too many women are falsely reassured because it doesn't hurt). I did think about cancer, but it didn't hurt, so I didn't rush to see about it right away. But I did mention it on my next appointment with the doctor."

"And when was that, Mrs Foster?" " I saw Dr Carter about a month or so later. I still didn't worry about it being a cancer. He checked me and then he got all excited and started fussing about women carrying around these cancers for years before telling anybody. But he never told me I should be checking myself. How was I to know?"

"I understand. But now you can pass the word to your friends about the importance of checking themselves regularly."

"Tha's right and I do just that. I had my surgery in, I think, 1972, and I'm doing fine. I have a little swelling in my arm but it don't bother me too bad. I can still do all my work and we still go fishin'just about every weekend."

"That's wonderful. You've done very well, Mrs Foster. Now here's another question for somebody. Did any of your doctors sit down and explain other choices of treatment? Mrs Robinson—Peggy?"

"Well, no. My doctor just said what had to be done and I went along with it. I figured he would know best", said Mrs Robinson.

"I already told you I didn't even know my breast was going to be removed for sure, much less any other possible choices", said Peggy.

"Okay. Peggy, you and Mrs Foster have told us about your husbands' reactions to your surgery. What about you, Mrs Robinson? How did your husband respond?"

It didn't hurt, so I didn't rush to see about it right away.

My doctor just said what had to be done and I went along with it. I figured he would know best
•••••••

My husband was left in the dark, more or less. He always felt the surgeon avoided talking to him or felt awkward about keeping him informed. Maybe it was because he was a white doctor. We were never told about reconstructive surgery and the doctor never said too much about practical things such as using padded bras or suggest the best way to dress. I think he left it up to the people in rehabilitation and the American Cancer Society ladies that visit after surgery to fill me in on those things. But I learned a lot. At least I know how to pronounce 'prosthesis', now.

"Anyway, we were referred back to my personal doctor, but my husband and I both wished the surgeon himself had gone over all these things and gave us more attention and advice. After all, he wasn't too busy to cut off my breast."

Apparently Mrs Robinson didn't understand the team approach to medical care. In the old days the doctor carried most of the responsibility. **Today**, the doctor depends on agencies and health workers, and delegates many tasks. But the doctor must be sure the patient understands this team approach.

Mrs Robinson continued, "After my operation, we weren't able to sit down and talk more than five minutes with the surgeon. He never seemed to have time. I made a list of things to ask because he rushed me. At least I thought he did. Even with a list I couldn't get my questions answered. My family doctor told me to call the surgeon if I had any problems. So there you are. I just wish doctors would take a little more time with their patients."

Some things for **some** patients cannot be delegated. The doctor must understand that too.

"Well, let me voice my view on this. Only a few years ago most physicians, including myself, felt a

BREAST CANCER / BLACK WOMAN   13

strong responsibility in making the decisions on a particular line of treatment. After all, the patient had no means of judging what was the best treatment; and we believed the patient depended on our guidance. So you must take that into consideration when you tell me that your doctors left you in the dark. Perhaps, if he had spelled out all the options and all the types of procedures and treatments and all the possible complications you would be so confused you'd still be in the dark."

Over the past twenty years things have changed dramatically. Today, in 1993, there is more information available to the public than ever before, and patients can learn about various diagnostic methods and treatment options. Certainly every patient has the right to ask questions and participate in therapy decisions.

Now, we have what they call peer review, where doctors monitor the work of their fellow doctors; and there's quality assurance, where doctors and ordinary citizens monitor the activities of doctors. These committees are set up to assure better care and communication between doctor and patient.

Doctors must keep up with new innovations and treatments through continuing medical education and in some cases re-certification. These are all forces that have affected the doctor-patient relationship and the physician must respond to these new constraints and keep the patient and family fully informed or find himself isolated in a precarious position.

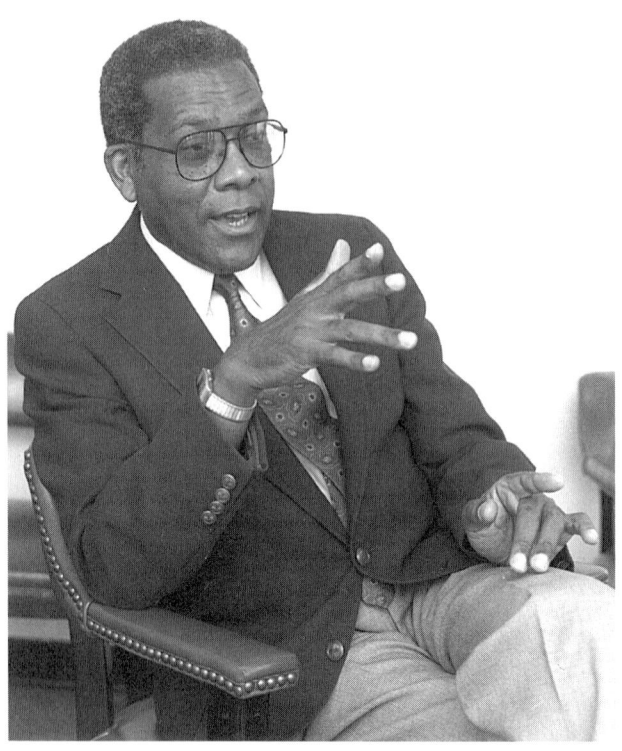

Certainly every patient has the right to ask questions and participate in therapy decisions. Doctors must keep up with new innovations and treatments through continuing medical education and in some cases re-certification. These are all forces that have affected the doctor-patient relationship and the physician must respond to these new constraints and keep the patient and family fully informed.

> *I still think the doctor should explain more", said Peggy. Doctor Johnson, patients just want to know what's happening. That's all.*
> ● ● ● ● ● ● ●

"I still think the doctor should explain more", said Peggy. Doctor Johnson, patients just want to know what's happening. That's all."

"You're right. Now let's see what's next. Oh yes. Did any of you have a visit from someone from the American Cancer Society?"

"Let me tell you about the women from the American Cancer Society, Doctor."

"Yes, the Reach to Recovery Program. Did they visit you Peggy? Was it worthwhile?"

"In a way, I believe it was. I was feeling so bad I needed a shoulder to cry on or at least someone to talk to. Like I said, my husband was out to lunch and my doctor was out in space. But the Reach to Recovery program helped. The person from the American Cancer Society was very nice. She told me about where to get a bra and who to call to compare different styles. She gave me a little pillow to wear in my bra when I was discharged from the hospital. You'd be surprised to know how important it is to have some kind of padding in your bra just to get home from the hospital."

"Did you get a visitor from the American Cancer Society, Mrs Foster?"

"My lady came by and we had a good visit too. She was real polite and told me she was from the American Cancer Society and had had the same operation and was doing fine; and she left me some little folders to read."

"Was she a black woman, Mrs Foster?" "Yes. I think she was about my age too. We talked about families and grandchildren and such. She showed me pictures. And you know, we knew some of the same people. In fact I'd been to her church to a musical program. I talked with her several times after I got home."

Mrs Robinson chimed in, "Those ladies from the American Cancer Society were nice to me too, Doctor Johnson, but some of those nurses and aides I had in the hospital were horrible."

"Tell us about that, Mrs Robinson?" "Do you know, they let me lay there and suffer. I could hear 'em laughing and talking down at their station. Wouldn't answer my buzzer for nothing, and when they did, they'd just leave me for hours before I got a pain shot. And I thought some of them were just too rough when changing my dressing or getting me to walk. Of course they say they have to be rough to get patients to do for themselves. But that's not true, because some other nurses were just as sweet and got me to exercise and walk just as much. I believe some nurses are just cruel and need to suffer themselves before they're allowed to wait on patients. This goes for white **and** black nurses"

"Of course when we're sick we may be more sensitive and perhaps more demanding, but still there may be some truth in what you say. I know I'm a lot more understanding of a patient with a back sprain, since I sprained by own back.

"I've always felt that black patients expect more out of black nurses, because they identify with them— black and female. They look for those nurturing characteristics found in grandmothers and mothers who cared for them through childhood sicknesses. I've been hospitalized more than once myself. Believe me even a half-mean nurse (black, white, Asian, or whatever) is a total disaster for a patient in pain.

"Okay now. Someone tell me about how you made out around the house. How'd you cope with going back to work? Let's see now. Mrs Foster, you had your mastectomy in 1972. Tell us about your rehabilita-

> *My husband and I talked a little about plastic surgery, We decided not to have any more surgery.*
> • • • • • • •

tion. Did you have any complications?"

"Well not too much. My arm and hand stayed real swoll' for a few weeks, my shoulder was stiff and o' course my chest hurt for a long time; but I kept workin' it and wearing that elastic sleeve and eventually everything got better. But I still use an elastic sleeve to keep down the swelling."

"What about follow-up visits to your doctor?" "Well I saw my doctor every month for a long time." "Did he seem attentive and understanding?" "Yes he did. He wasn't the one that operated. He was just my family doctor, but he watched over me pretty good I think. I'm supposed to go back every six months to get a check on my other breast and get an x-ray."

"Do you recall anything about the hospital and nursing staff." "Yes. They all seemed real good. I didn't have no trouble." "What about going back to work or just resuming your daily activities? Did anyone have trouble coping with that? What about you, Mrs Robinson?"

"That part was just fine", said Mrs Robinson. "My family was real supportive. My husband and I talked a little about plastic surgery, but the mastectomy hasn't seemed to interfere with our sexual relations and I had no problem with my clothes fitting okay, since I used the prosthesis in my bra. We decided not to have any more surgery. I didn't work outside the home, so I didn't have to worry about going out every day to a job."

"And you Peggy. You were working. How did things go when you returned to work?"

"At that time I was working in an insurance office as a clerk. A great big room with umpteen desks and women wall to wall, typewriters, and phones buzzing for eight hours straight. I just felt awkward. Like ev-

> *It was a pretty good job, but I just up and quit. Everybody just acted differently after my surgery.*
> • • • • • • •

erybody was looking at me. My doctor told me that plastic surgery couldn't be done in my case, and I was always aware that so much of my chest was gone—not just my breast, but muscles too. I just felt like people were looking through my clothes.

"It was a pretty good job, but I just up and quit. Everybody just acted differently after my surgery. Somebody would ask me every day how I felt. You know how folks are when they're trying to be nice?"

"Everybody was just too polite all the time. Or else someone wanted to let me know that they knew someone who had breast cancer and how brave they were until the end."

"They did me that way too chile", said Mrs Foster. Look like I couldn't go to church without some well meanin' soul asking me if I was doin' okay. And do you know people be telling me I looked tired.

I declare people don't know **what** to say. Now that bothered me more'n anything. If the shoe was on the other foot, I believe it'd be a different story."

"Amen to that."

REFERENCES

1. Incidence of breast cancer (response to letter).JNCI 80:2, 1988

2. Kern KA: Causes of Breast Cancer Malpractice Litigation: A 20-year civil court review. Arch Surg 127:542-547, 1992

3. Bagle J Burnette C: The effects of breast cancer disclosure legislation on physician disclosure practices [disertation]. Baltimore, The Johns Hopkins University, 1989

In 54% of black women diagnosed with breast cancer, the cancer has already spread. Compare this to white patients. In 48 % of white women the cancer has already spread when first diagnosed. In 11% of black women breast cancer has metastasized widely; but in only 7% of white women has cancer already spread widely when first seen. The incidence of breast cancer is highest among both black and white women in the highest socio-economic and educational levels. But women at the lower socio-economic level are diagnosed at later stages and generally fare worse with treatment. These women, disproportionately black, need greater emphasis in screening initiatives.

Wells BL, Horm JW American Journal of Public Health 82:1383-1385, 1992

Black women are less likely to have routine breast examinations. There is a definite differential in access to health care services and mammography. As a result, black women when first diagnosed are 2 times more likely to have Stage IV breast cancer and 1 1/2 times more likely to have Stage III cancer than white women. Black women are only half as likely to have Stage I cancer; and black women are twice as likely to have a tumor over two inches in diameter when first seen. These findings put black women at special risk.

Coates RJ, Bransfield DD, Wesley M, et al Black/White cancer survival study group; Journal National Cancer Institute 84:938-950 1992

CHAPTER TWO

WHERE IT ALL BEGINS
Breast Development, Construction and Function

*I*t was *HEALTH AWARENESS DAY* at a predominantly black inner city community center. The event had been well publicized and the sponsors were happy with the turnout. The Public Health Department, The Commission on Aging and several other agencies were represented with booths and brochures. Purveyors of medical information had descended en masse to deliver the message of caution and emphasize the virtue of personal health. Young people were being inundated with the dangers of drug abuse, AIDS, and sexually transmitted diseases. Older folks were getting their blood pressure checked, and lining up for cholesterol testing. It was all about making good choices, and respecting the mind and body. There were posters about diabetes, nutrition, and sickle-cell anemia.

The organizers also planned to cover topics on cancer, especially lung cancer and breast cancer. Lung cancer was a preventable disease, so the dangers of cigarette smoking would be highlighted with videos and talk sessions and hand-outs.

I was invited to say a few words on breast cancer, since that was an area of special interest to me; and the local chapter of the American Cancer Society was helpful in providing a film on breast cancer that emphasized early detection. I had decided to give a brief talk on the anatomy and function of the breast before showing the film. I was ushered to a small auditorium seating about 350 people. From the rostrum I had a chance to glance over the audience.

There were mostly women, of all ages. Some holding small children. Towards the rear of the room I spied a large group of boys and girls—teenagers, laughing and noisy and just being teenagers. A sea of precocious youth, mostly black, bursting at the seams with energy and life.

Then I was being introduced. "We are happy to welcome Dr Johnson to this segment of HEALTH AWARENESS DAY. He's going to speak on..."

While the introduction continued I had a chance to look at my notes and I took a moment to study the faces before me—a few dull and distracted; but most seemed interested or at least curious. The youth in the rear seemed more interested in each other with all the chatter and gum popping. Only a few seemed to be interested in what I had to say. Surely, I thought, some would be curious enough to listen in spite of the distractions around them. Who knows? One of these youngsters amid the confusion may one day discover some universal truth that would make a difference.

"....So let's give Dr Johnson your attention." I stepped to the lectern and began to speak.

"As part of HEALTH AWARENESS DAY, we've been invited to discuss various health issues with you.

I stepped to the lectern and began to speak . . ."The good news is that over 85 percent of breast cancers can be cured if found early."

> *Too many black women are lost to breast cancer because so many are unaware of the danger signals and too few are being checked on a regular basis.*
>
> ● ● ● ● ● ●

You've been learning about sexually transmitted disease and AIDS and sickle-cell anemia and other health issues. Well, in this segment the topic is breast cancer, one of the major cancers—affecting one in eight women in this country.

"My presentation, the movie and handouts, will be stressing the same thing—your responsibility to protect your health and the health of your family. So it's important that you know something about breast cancer, by far the number one cancer in American women.

"The good news is that over 85 percent of breast cancers can be cured if found early. The bad news is that relatively more black women are likely to die of breast cancer. Does anyone have any idea why that is so?"

No one responded. Faces were blank. But the question at least quieted the room and even the teenagers were glancing my way. I continued.

"Too many black women are lost to breast cancer because so many are unaware of the danger signals and too few are being checked on a regular basis.

"Now before we view the movie from the American Cancer Society about the danger signals and early detection, let me review some basics. Let's go back to where it all begins. Let's examine the normal anatomy and function of the breast."

"First, we'll look at the breast through the microscope, so to speak, and examine the various tissues that make up the human breast, such as the glandular structure, the lymph channels, the blood vessels and the underlying muscles. Then we shall review how body hormones affect the normal breast and, in some cases, stimulate cancerous growth. Now relax. I'm not going to try to impress you with high sounding medical words. We'll keep things simple and understandable. And please feel free to ask questions as we go along.

"By way of introduction I shall make a few remarks about the breast development in various animals, and then outline the growth and development of the breast in humans. I have plenty of copies of the presentation for you to take for further study."

Mammals and Breast Tissue:

Warm blooded animals that have specialized glands that produce milk are called mammals and those milk-producing glands are called mammary glands. Before birth a continuous thickened ridge develops in the skin along the right and left sides of the embryo's chest and abdomen. From Figure 2-1 you can see that these so-called milk ridges are paired and extend from high on the chest wall to the groin. Later, paired milk glands appear along these ridges. In the cat and dog we find six or seven paired glands developing. A similar arrangement is also found in the pig, the rabbit and a wide variety of other mammals. Some mam-

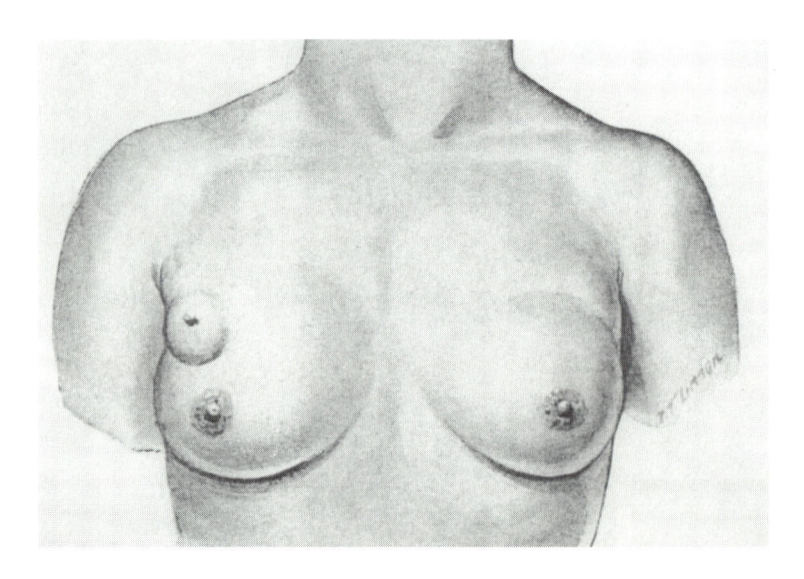

Fig. 2-1
THE MILK RIDGES. The broken lines represent the position of the milk ridges that are very prominent in the embryo. A nipple and breast tissue may form anywhere along these ridges.

Fig. 2-2
A RUDIMENTARY NIPPLE. An undeveloped nipple is present. Occasionally this breast is functional, but there are no reports of cancer developing in this immature breast tissue.

Fig. 2-3
THE GLANDS OF THE BREAST.
The breast is made up of glandular tissue surrounded and supported by fatty tissue and thin suspensory ligaments. Glandular tissue is made up of acini in the periphery where milk is produced. Hundreds of acini converge to form lobules. Lobules converge to form 10 to 20 lobes which form ducts that empty at the nipple. Cancer develops in the ducts, lobes, and lobules—but mostly in the ducts. As the breast ages the suspensory ligaments lengthen and the glandular tissue atrophies and the breast is less dense. This allows physical examination and x-rays to find cancers much more easily in older women.

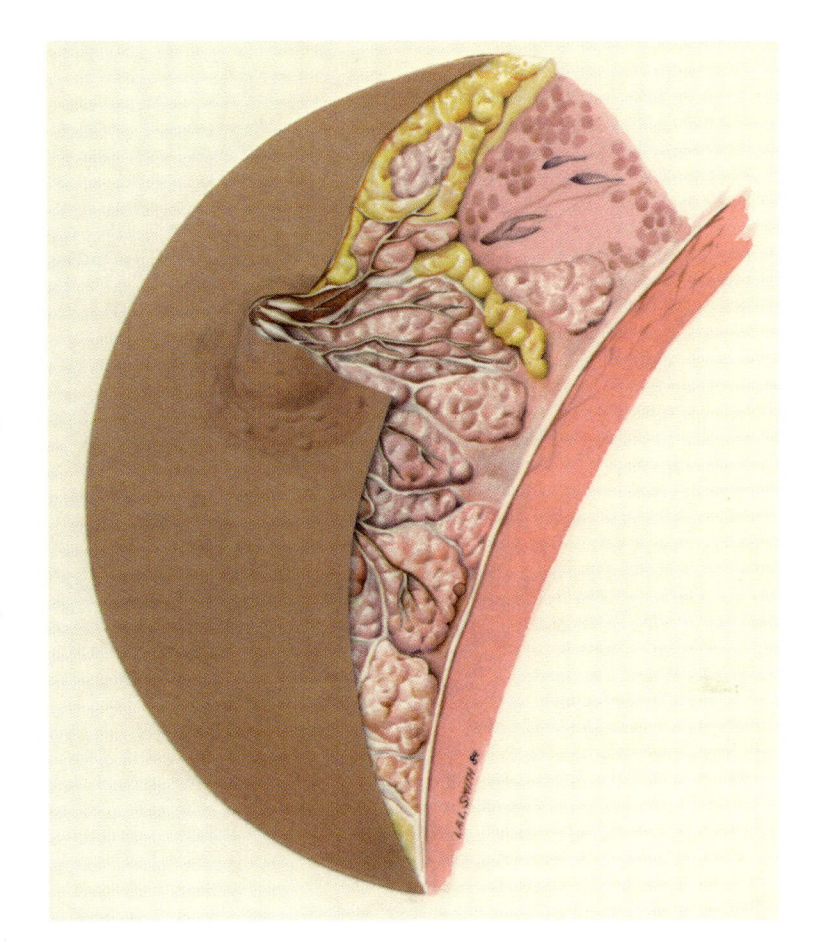

mals show a lack of development of the complete milk ridge with milk glands developing only on the chest or only on the abdomen. Paired mammary glands are found only in the abdominal region in the cow, the goat, the whale and the lion. Single paired milk glands evolve in the pectoral or chest area in such animals as the elephant, the walrus, and members of the ape family.

The milk ridges that unfold in the human fetus gradually fade long before birth, leaving a pair of budding mammary glands on the pectoral or chest area. Occasionally the milk ridge persists in a rudimentary form along the lower chest and even on the abdomen. This gives rise to undeveloped nipples and, rarely, even functioning breast tissue. Hence, one may discover an incidental atrophic nipple in the lower chest or upper abdomen in a man or woman, that is, for the most part, of little consequence (Figure 2-2).

Among the family of mammals, breast cancer is found most often in the human. It very rarely occurs spontaneously in the rat and dog; but it is found in no other mammalian creature. Through chemicals and breeding, breast cancer can be easily produced in the laboratory rat; and in this way cancer can be studied.

Glandular Structure:

The breast is divided into 15 to 20 lobes, radially positioned about the nipple as seen in Figure 2-3. These lobes in turn are sectioned into lobules which in turn are formed by hundreds of acini, which are the basic units that secrete milk. Channels that drain the acini, lobules and lobes converge at the nipple as ducts. Each duct has its own separate set of lobes, lobules and acini; and a copious layer of fat separates the lobules and surrounds the developing breast tissue.

Blood and Lymphatic Supply:

A maze of blood vessels feeds into the breast tissue. See Figure 2-4. Estrogen hormones from the ovary regulate circulation to the breast by dilating the arteries and veins. These blood vessels, especially veins, serve as pathways for cancer spread and evidence suggests that cancer is already seeding into the circulation long before the primary tumor can be palpated. However, if the body is not overwhelmed, the immune system is able to destroy these

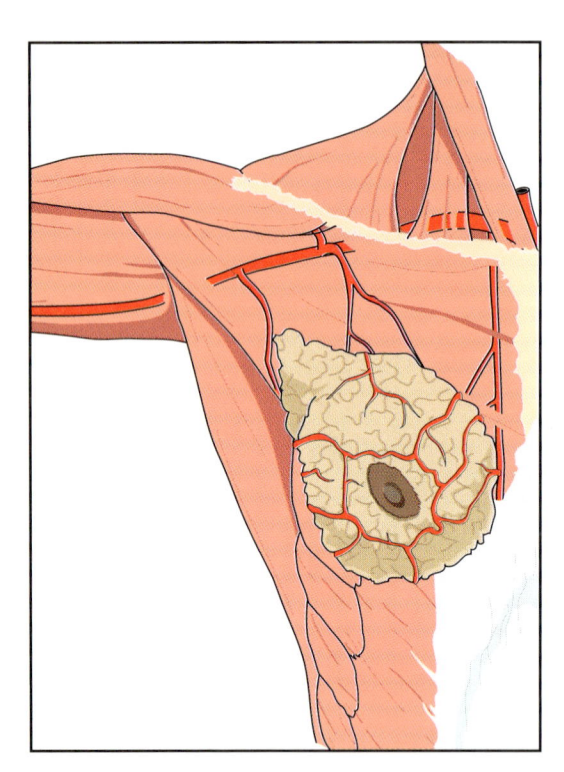

Fig. 2-4
THE ARTERIES OF THE BREAST. The arterial supply is very elaborate spreading out as a network over the entire breast. Under the influence of female hormones the blood supply increases remarkably. During pregnancy more blood vessels open up to service the enlarged and engorged breast.

early malignant cells.

Another important network that provides channels for cancer spread is the lymphatic system seen in Figure 2-5. The lymphatic vessels are much like veins but so thin-walled that they are generally invisible to the naked eye. Consequently, one may tend to forget their importance.

But in our anatomical road map these lymph channels are the **major** route allowing cancer cells to spread into deeper structures called lymph nodes. Therefore we must have a clear idea where these lymph nodes are located and be able to examine them for enlargement and tenderness. The lymph nodes that drain the breast are clustered, for the most part, in the axilla, or arm pit. One must carefully palpate the axilla along with the breast for suspicious irregularities and tenderness.

The lymph channels ordinarily contain a clear fluid, that is nothing more than blood without the red blood cells. They are as plentiful as the capillaries and represent a vital part of the circulation. Blood, except for the red cells, seeps into these lymph channels and eventually this circulatory fluid is strained by lymph nodes, and eventually is returned to the general circulation. The lymph nodes are an important link in our defense system against cancer spread and cancer cells are trapped in the lymph nodes where many are destroyed. But some cells eventually escape the lymph nodes and are carried further until finally they empty into the general circulation and are then carried to such places as the lungs, liver and brain.

As mentioned above, the majority of lymph nodes

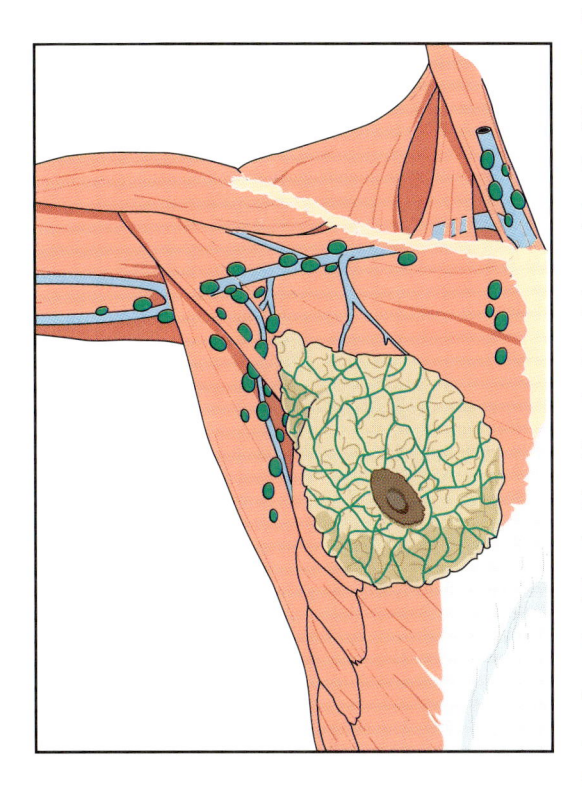

Fig. 2-5
VEINS AND LYMPH CHANNELS OF THE BREAST.
Veins and Lymph channels (in green) are laced throughout the breast, chest wall, and into the axilla (armpit). Lymph channels drain lymph fluid to regional lymph nodes (in green) mostly in the axilla. The lymph nodes eventually drain into the blood stream. The lymph channels and veins are the main routes by which cancer spreads from the breast to the armpit and then to other parts of the body.

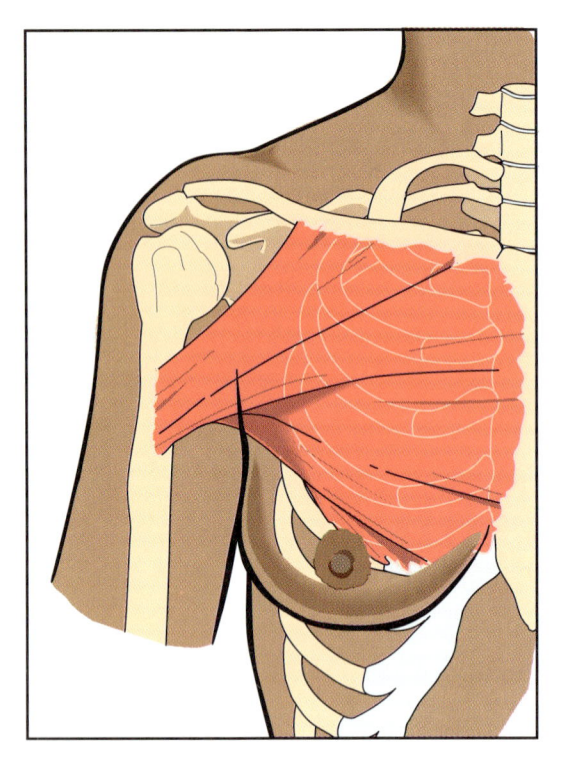

Fig. 2-6
MUSCLES UNDER THE BREAST. The muscles under the breast include the Pectoralis Major which is shown. The Pectoralis Minor is hidden underneath the Pectoralis Major. These muscles are almost never removed nowadays when operating for breast cancer. In fact if cancer is found early, the breast itself can be spared in most cases, with excellent results. If your doctor says you need radical surgery that includes removal of the muscles, get another opinion.

that drain the breast are found nestled in the armpit; and consequently, the major flow of cancer cells from the breast by way of the lymphatics is laterally towards the axilla (armpit). It is these groups of nodes that you and your physician will be carefully checking for enlargement and tenderness. **Any non-tender mass in the breast with a firm nodule in the axilla demands immediate investigation for cancer.**

However, lymph nodes in the axilla may also be enlarged and painful if there is infection in the breast or local infection in the axilla, or even in the arm or distal hand. A common occurrence is a minor skin infection in a hair follicle in the armpit with an associated enlarged node.

Muscles Under the Breast:

There are two important muscles underlying the breast: The pectoralis major and the pectoralis minor noted in Figure 2-6. They are significant because cancer cells can migrate directly into the muscle tissue or travel by way of lymphatic channels to lymph nodes that lie between the muscles.

The pectoralis major lies immediately under the breast and fat layer. It originates along the margin of the sternum (breast bone) medially and clavicle (collar bone) above. A few slips spring from the rib cage below. The muscle then sweeps laterally across the chest wall to insert as a fibrous band into the humerus (arm bone) tucked under the deltoid shoulder muscle.

The pectoralis achieves its greatest development in

28 WHERE IT ALL BEGINS

the bird family where it becomes the highly specialized, powerful muscle of flight.

If this muscle is removed during cancer surgery it may cause only slight functional impairment. However, the deformity is very significant.

The pectoralis minor is a much smaller muscle that lies beneath the pectoralis major. It helps to stabilize the shoulder in concert with other muscles and if surgically removed there is no appreciable loss of function; but again, it adds to the deformity.

The mutilation of radical surgery with removal of the pectoralis muscles has been replaced by more conservative procedures. If the cancer is discovered in time, in many instances the breast need not be removed. Only the cancer itself is excised along with some lymph nodes from the armpit.

Hormone Control of Human Breast Tissue:

At birth the male and female breasts are essentially the same. The nipples are inverted and the surrounding coin-shaped skin, the areola, is slightly pigmented. Then a few days after birth, the areola darkens, nipples evert and the breast tissue swells in about 70 percent of newborns. Half of these babies will then secrete a cloudy fluid called "witch's milk". These changes are due to the influence of estrogen flowing into the child from the mother's blood stream by way of the placenta. But in two to three weeks after birth these changes will subside and the child's breast will ease into a resting stage. Breast tissue in both sexes will remain in a similar state of repose for years—until the awakening at puberty.

As puberty dawns, about age ten to twelve, all sorts of transformations begin to take place. Little children begin sprouting like weeds. Acne starts popping out.

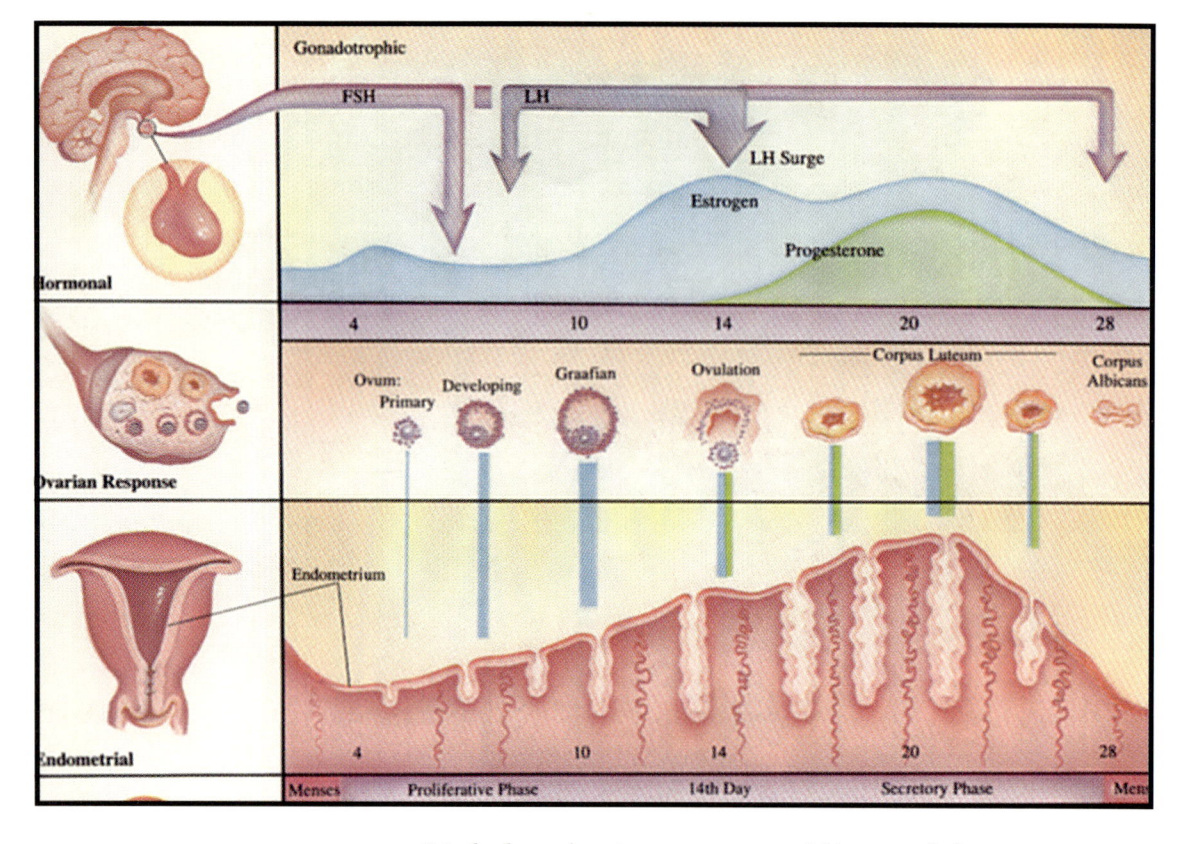

Fig. 2-7
FEMALE HORMONES. The menstrual cycle averages 28 days. During the first half of the cycle estrogen causes a build up of the lining of the womb. The lining is then thickened and develops more blood vessels as the result of progesterone. When the production of these female hormones decrease, menstruation takes place. During the latter part of the cycle just before menstruation, the breast has enlarged by 50 per cent under the influence of these hormones. It is believed that estrogen is a factor in the development of breast cancer.

Little boys' voices start crackling and deepening into maturity. Pubic and axillary hair growth and muscular development are a part of this process. Little girls begin to snicker and talk about "boys"; and boys start looking at budding girls in a different way. Dating and dancing and going steady are a normal progression.

Ovaries have matured to the point that they can respond to the follicle stimulating hormone (FSH) produced by the pituitary gland located at the base of the brain. From the diagram in Figure 2-7, you can see that FSH hormone induces the ovary to form follicles which in turn produce estrogens. As the estrogen level rises even higher in the early teen years, ovaries begin to produce eggs, and the menstrual cycle begins. The estrogens are responsible for all the female characteristics, such as the high pitched voice, distribution of fat, shape of the pelvis, the smooth

Fig. 2-8
BREAST DEVELOPMENT: CHILD-ADOLESCENT-ADULT. The breast in preadolescent boys and girls is essentially the same. At adolescence under sexual hormone influence the breast begins to increase in volume in both boys and girls. The small lump in the boys' breast subsides in a few weeks. The enlarging breast in the adolescent girl, under the influence of estrogen continues to the fully developed adult female breast with a full complement of lobes and ducts.

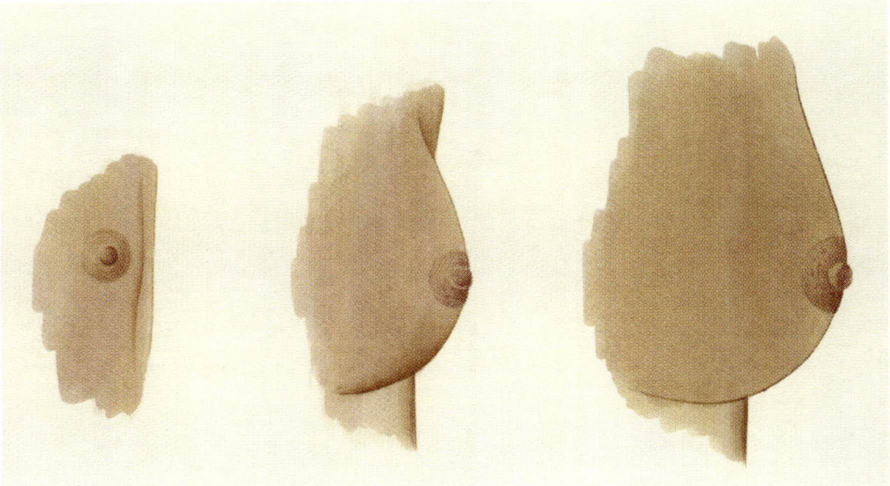

face, and, of course, the maturation of the breast.

In the pre-teen years enough estrogens cause a swelling under the nipple called the prepubertal bud. As the breast begins to protrude, glandular tissue spreads out in a fairly uniform circular manner and in a few short years the general contour of the young adult female breast is attained. See Figure 2-8.

During the first three to seven days of the menstrual cycle there is vaginal bleeding, or active menstrual flow as depicted in Figure 2-7. This corresponds to a temporary low level of estrogen production. When estrogen is at a low level, the lining of the uterus or womb cannot be maintained and it is shed as menstrual flow.

About the seventh day of the cycle, new levels of estrogen are gradually being secreted by the ovary under the influence of the FSH from the pituitary gland.

When the estrogen blood level reaches a certain point the lining of the uterus can be maintained and menstruation ceases. The lining continues to thicken for the next seven to ten days. The estrogen buildup also affects the breasts. There is a fifty percent increase in volume. The breasts become firm and occasionally tender. At this stage a tumor or cancer may be easily missed during physical examination. That's why your doctor will tell you to examine your

BREAST CANCER / BLACK WOMAN

breasts a few days after the menstrual period ceases.

About the fourteenth day, or mid-cycle, the follicle produces an egg which travels by way of the Fallopian tube to the lining of the uterus already prepared by estrogen stimulation. Refer again to Figure 2-7. At the same time the high level of estrogen inhibits the flow of FSH from the pituitary and stimulates the pituitary gland to secrete the luteinizing hormone (LH) which acts on the ruptured follicle to produce progesterone. Progesterone is needed to further develop the lining of the uterus to make it hospitable and able to nourish the egg should it become impregnated. Towards the end of the cycle the rising tide of progesterone inhibits the LH from the pituitary which in turn causes a fall of progesterone.

By this time both progesterone and estrogen are at a low ebb and the uterine lining can no longer be maintained. Consequently menstrual flow begins anew as the lining of the uterus is shed.

Should pregnancy take place, the ovaries continue to supply the estrogen hormone in even larger volume and one of the major target organs, the breast, responds by growth and elaboration of the lobes and lobules. There is marked engorgement and enlargement of 2 to 3 times the resting state and pigmentation of the areola deepens and spreads to the adjacent breast skin. Veins dilate and stretch marks appear. After delivery and cessation of pregnancy, the hormone prolactin is released from the pituitary and combined with the action of a suckling baby, the breast produces a flow of milk that is maintained so long as suckling continues, even up to 36 months or longer. After milk production has ended, the breast proceeds to a resting state. Following childbirth, breast tissue is less dense and cancers can be discovered more readily by palpation. If a breast mass is found during pregnancy, mammography is delayed until the final month or so of the pregnancy. Ultrasound can be used to detect whether the mass is a cyst. There is no contraindication of removing a mass under local anesthesia during pregnancy.

At the time of the menopause, in response to further lowering of estrogen, the breast atrophies and is replaced by fat. The contour becomes even more lax and small cancers can then be more easily palpated and seen on x-ray.

———

"Now then, are there any questions or comments before we show the movie on breast cancer detection? Yes young man, what is your question?"

A tall gangling youth awkwardly stood up in the back of the room and asked, "What about men? Do men get breast cancer too?'

After the giggling died down (teenagers laugh about almost anything) I spoke. "What's your name?'

"Amos Wilson." "Yes Amos, it's true. Men **do** get breast cancer, but it is extremely rare. It's so rare that most of the time no one thinks that a sore or lump in the male breast is a cancer until it has spread and is probably incurable. So men must also be on the lookout for themselves as well as the women in their lives.

"But the most common cancer today in black men is lung cancer and almost all of it can be prevented by not smoking. You don't smoke do you Amos?"

Amos smiled and the teenagers snickered. "Thank you everyone for your attention. This overview that I've presented is intended to answer some basic questions about the structure and function of the breast. I hope that it will also serve as a focal point for additional questions that you may wish to discuss at home or with your family doctor. You know, if you have a better understanding of where breast cancer begins you should be able to appreciate your role in detecting breast cancer and warning others of the danger signals."

As we shall see in the next chapter, detecting breast cancer early is the best way to control and cure.

CHAPTER THREE

A CASE FOR SHERLOCK HOLMES
Making the Diagnosis

For a hundred years we've observed and admired Sherlock Holmes as he deciphered many baffling mysteries with his unique brand of expertise. The detective would methodically sift the clues and meticulously dissect each case using his fine sense of inductive reasoning. What seemed at first glance to be a string of disconnected facts would be dramatically interwoven into a pattern of logic and order. Finally, to our utter astonishment, Holmes would take us through the maze of clues that eventually pointed to the guilty party. His assistant, the befuddled Dr Watson, would finally raise his eyebrows and exclaim, "By jove Holmes, you're right".

In the same way the fictional character Sherlock Holmes demonstrated his talent for solving mysteries, health workers and patients in the real world must pool their talent and determination to solve the breast cancer mystery that confronted over 150,000 newly diagnosed women in 1990, and another 183,000 new cases in 1993.

Indeed, the pursuit, the diagnosis, and the treatment of breast cancer is medical detective work of a high order. Many characters are involved and all play essential parts—research workers, physicians, hospital personnel, and the patient herself.

It can not be emphasized enough that **every woman must assume full partnership in detecting breast cancer.** This means awareness and knowing the warning signs. This is absolutely crucial in detecting the breast cancer villain before irretrievable damage is done. The doctor's training and the tools of medicine can only work effectively when the cancer criminal is not ignored or sheltered, but promptly exposed for effective elimination.

It has been reported that more than 90 percent of breast cancers are detected by the patient (this figure may be decreasing with increased use of routine mammography).[1] In some cases a minor injury may prompt a woman to examine the breast and thus discover the lump. The problem is that these tumors are often reported after the cancer has spread. The National Cancer Institute survey in 1971 reported that in 68 percent of new cases among black women breast cancer had already metastasized when first diagnosed; however, in only 58 percent of white women had the spread of cancer already occurred when first seen.[2] There is no question that the chance for cure decreases precipitously if there is spread at the time of first discovery. Cure rate for cancer confined to the breast should be 80 percent or more. This excellent prognosis quickly falls to a 25 to 50 percent survival if the cancer has metastasized when first uncovered.

Consequently, beginning about age twenty, every young woman should begin the habit of checking her breasts monthly to detect unusual nodules.[3]

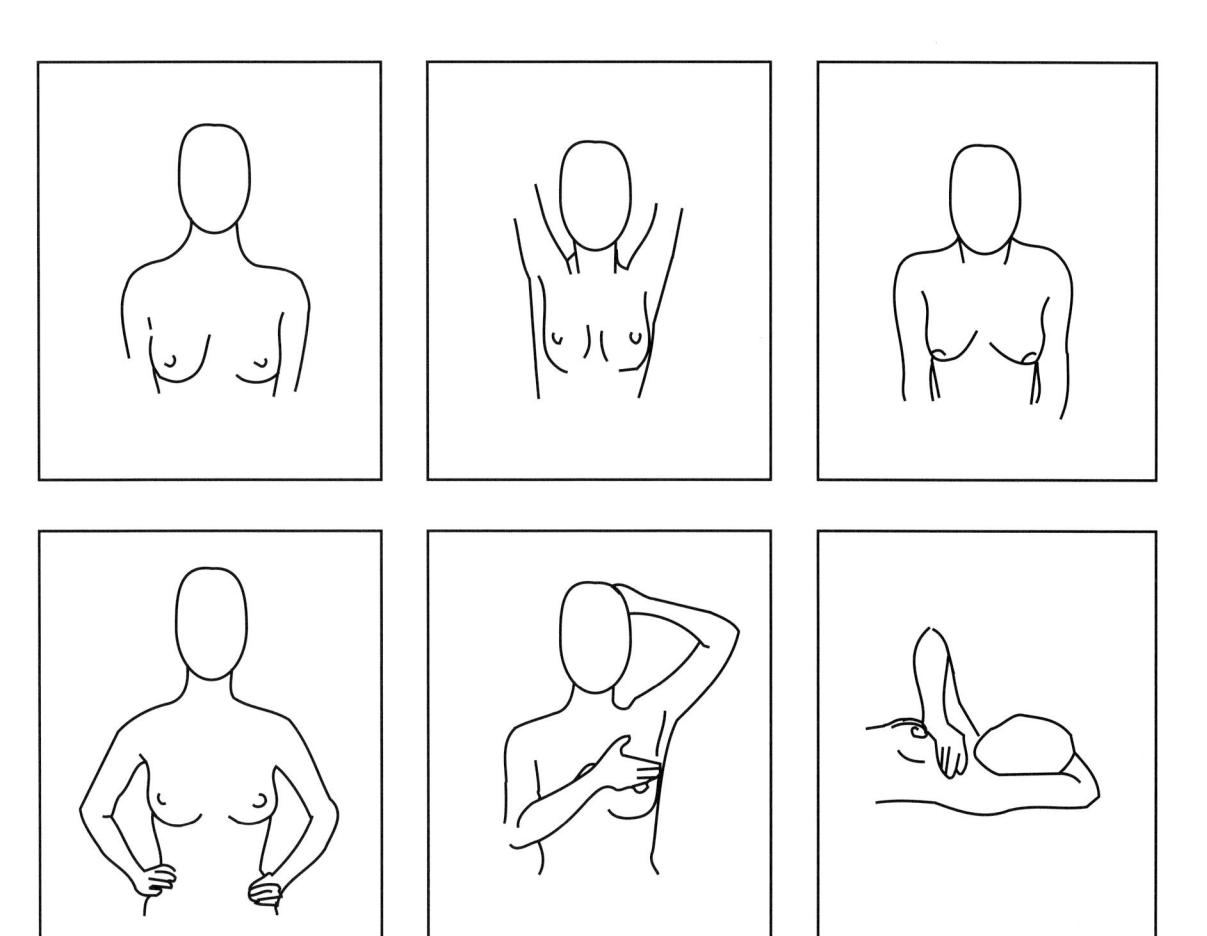

Fig. 3-1
BREAST SELF EXAMINATION (BSE).
Monthly BSE beginning at age twenty should continue on a regular basis for a lifetime. See text.

It is especially important for young black women since they have breast cancer one and a half times the rate of white women before age thirty-five.

BREAST SELF EXAMINATION

Early diagnosis is the general thrust of Breast Self-Examination (BSE) spearheaded by the American Cancer Society. Studies have shown that regular BSE, a simple maneuver to master, can actually save lives.[3] A physician or other trained health provider can guide you through the various steps as you learn to examine your own breast. Also there are instructive brochures available at all American Cancer Society Units across the country. Although the exact procedure proposed may vary somewhat among physicians, the general principles are the same. One should systematically search the breast for lumps or thickening on a regular monthly basis. This could be done about ten days after the menstrual flow begins each and every month. If there is no menstruation because of surgery or menopause then an exam on the same day each month seems to be adequate. The examination is divided between inspection and palpation.

Inspection: See Fig. 3-1. Stand before the mirror, chest exposed, and inspect the breasts looking for obvious deformity or irregularity. Notice superficial vein engorgement, skin dimpling or discoloration, or rash over the nipple area. Now lean forward. Again look in The mirror with a good light. Do both breasts move away from the chest wall in a similar manner or is there restrictions or dimpling not noticed before? Does either nipple appear to be pulled to one side or the other?

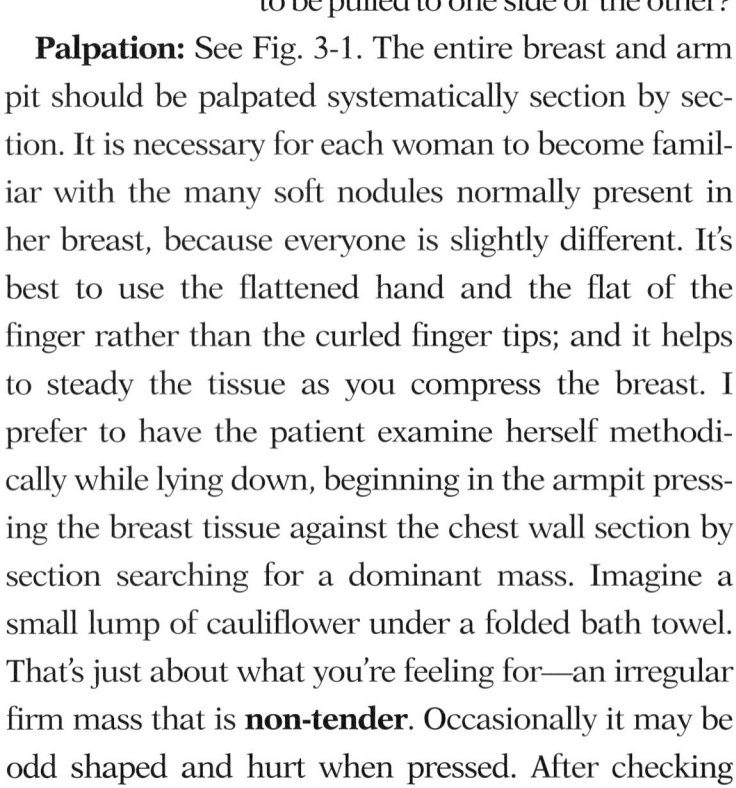

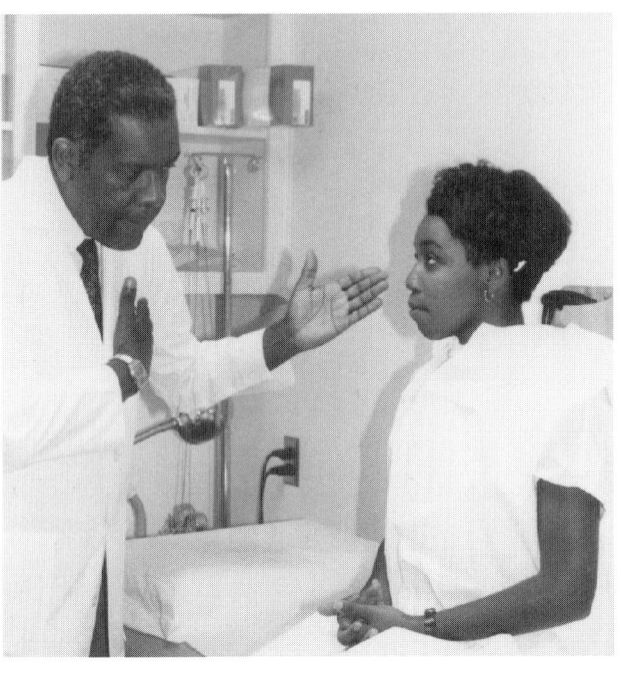

Palpation: See Fig. 3-1. The entire breast and arm pit should be palpated systematically section by section. It is necessary for each woman to become familiar with the many soft nodules normally present in her breast, because everyone is slightly different. It's best to use the flattened hand and the flat of the finger rather than the curled finger tips; and it helps to steady the tissue as you compress the breast. I prefer to have the patient examine herself methodically while lying down, beginning in the armpit pressing the breast tissue against the chest wall section by section searching for a dominant mass. Imagine a small lump of cauliflower under a folded bath towel. That's just about what you're feeling for—an irregular firm mass that is **non-tender**. Occasionally it may be odd shaped and hurt when pressed. After checking

Fig. 3-2
A PATIENT EXAMINES HER OWN BREAST WITH THE PHYSICIAN GIVING CAREFUL INSTRUCTION.
Every woman should be familiar with the soft normal nodularity of her own breast.

Cancer feels like a very hard knot that is usually not tender. Most cancers are found by the patient herself. In more than half of cancers found and reported by black women, the cancer has already spread. Therefore regular systematic BSE is crucial.

the breast a section at a time and finding no dominant lumps, you should gently compress the nipple between thumb and forefinger for evidence of blood or discharge. Thirty percent of women over the age of 60 with nipple discharge and no breast lump eventually prove to have breast cancer.

With monthly BSE you will soon **know** your normal nodularity and lumpiness. If there is any question, by all means, have your doctor go over it with you. Most breast lumps are either normal or represent benign disease. The chance of a lump being cancer increases with advancing years. Therefore, breast self examination is every bit as crucial as any detective insight your doctor can bring to bear on the case. According to the American Cancer Society only 25 percent of black women examine their breasts on a regular monthly basis. If breast cancer mortality is to be challenged successfully, not only must you engage in BSE regularly each month, but you must take it upon yourself to encourage all of your adult women friends to do likewise.

Periodically it is important to allow a physician or other trained health provider to examine the breast with you. Your questions and concerns should be discussed at that time. A yearly examination would seem adequate, and more frequent exams are warranted if a woman has certain risk factors. The American Cancer Society has explicit recommendations regarding the frequency of breast examination by a professional. We'll explore those guidelines in Chapter 5.

DIFFERENTIAL DIAGNOSIS

Once the breast lump is known to be present, the capable detective, like any worthy Sherlock Holmes,

Fig. 3-3
FIBROCYSTIC DYSPLASIA.
This is a very common condition among black women. Note the multiple dark round shadows in the x-ray that represent multiple cysts. These are often painful nodules, particularly a few days before the menses; but the discomfort can be controlled. Dysplasia generally improves and subsides after the menopause. This condition is associated with increased risk of breast cancer. If a nodule can not be distinguished from cancer then biopsy is imperative.

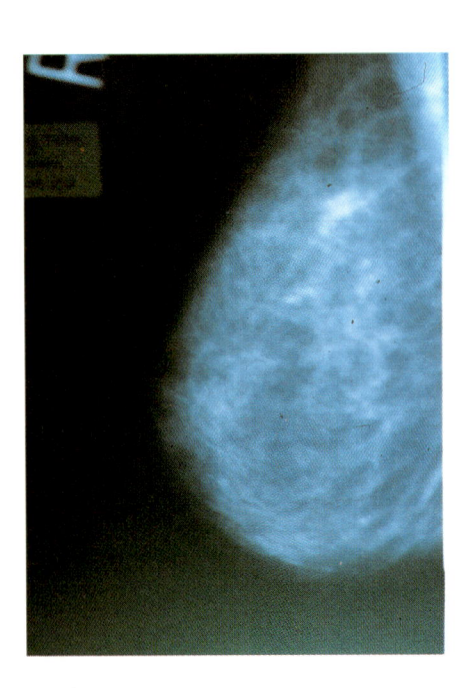

regards the mass as a prime suspect. The evidence must be tested, and conclusions drawn. Is this lump a cancer, a cyst or some benign interloper? What is the correct diagnosis among all the possibilities? Across the board only one in eight breast masses are actually cancer. This figure rises sharply in the older age groups. After age fifty, all breast lumps must be considered malignant until proven otherwise.

If the lump is not a cancer, what are the other possibilities? Several benign tumors come to mind. Your doctor will consider fibrocystic dysplasia, fibroadenoma, ductal papilloma, and fat necrosis. Let's briefly examine two of the more common benign problems that can be confused with cancer.

Fibrocystic Dysplasia

The most common tumor found in the breast between age 35 and the menopause is fibrocystic dysplasia, also called fibrocystic disease.[4] It manifests itself before the menopause as multiple nodules in both breasts. A single nodule may be quite prominent and the rest very small or not palpable. This may be impossible to distinguish from cancer and require aspiration, mammography (x-ray examination), and perhaps open biopsy.

After the menopause, estrogen hormone levels fall and fibrocystic dysplasia tends to soften and subside. At least one in seven women have this disease to some extent. Seldom does it cause significant discomfort, although occasionally the breasts may become taut and tender just before menstruation. A well-fitting brassiere can reduce the discomfort.

If the discomfort of fibrocystic dysplasia is not controlled by aspirin or other simple analgesics, then avoiding certain foods and medications that contain methylxanthine such as chocolate and certain asthma medications, is usually beneficial.

Methylxanthine is also found in coffee, tea, Anacin, Dristan, Midol and other medications commonly used. As a last resort, if the breast discomfort is unremitting, Vitamin E and androgen hormones can be used with good relief.[5] Most of the nodularity will disappear. If a dominant lump persists, then biopsy is imperative regardless of mammographic results.[6] Also it should be noted that since nicotine stimulates cystic formation, smoking cigarettes may contribute to fibrocystic dysplasia.

It is widely accepted that women with fibrocystic dysplasia have an increased risk of developing breast cancer, though recent studies in England have challenged this view.[7,8]

Although most of these benign nodules are solid and discrete some are confluent with neighboring nodules and some become cystic and fill with fluid. A diagnostic office procedure, transillumination, may be suggested by your doctor to show if the tumor is solid or cystic. It's quite probable that the medical detective will prefer a needle aspiration of the lump with the skin anesthetized. Many times a thin fluid, straw colored or pale greenish-gray, will be removed and the mass eliminated forever. The fluid is checked for cancer cells. If negative, the breast is simply observed for several months for possible recurrence of the cyst. If aspiration does not deflate the nodule it is assumed to be solid and if it is enlarging and fairly distinct from the other masses, a biopsy is mandatory to rule out cancer even if the mammogram does not suggest malignancy. It is true that the vast majority of cystic lesions tend to be

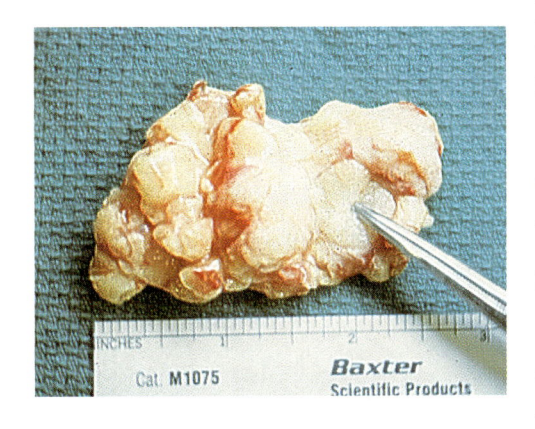

Fig. 3-4
BREAST BIOPSY OF FIBROCYSTIC DYSPLASIA. This tissue can not be differentiated from cancer by the naked eye. All tissue removed must be studied under the microscope to determine its true nature.

benign and indeed 90 percent are successfully handled by aspiration. If there is a recurrence of the same cyst after a second aspiration I would not hesitate to recommend surgical excision of the cyst even if the aspirate is negative for cancer cells.

If a woman is known to have fibrocystic dysplasia, it is **imperative** that breast self examination be done monthly about ten days after the menstrual period begins. A physician or other professional should examine the breast every six to eight months and a record kept for follow-up

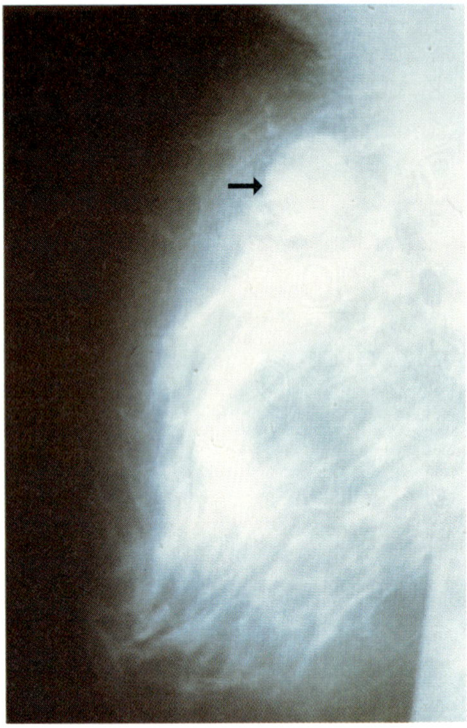

Fibroadenoma

This is a benign tumor that can only be distinguished from a cancer by microscopic examination.[9] Occasionally a number of these growths arise in the breast simultaneously. Often fibroadenoma is found as a single discrete freely movable tumor that is non-tender and when first discovered ranges in size from a peanut to a walnut. Some believe that estrogen stimulation is somehow causative because it grows rapidly during pregnancy when estrogen level is high, and birth control pills stimulate the rapid growth of fibroadenoma. It almost always develops in the young female—late teens or early twenties; in fact, it is the number one breast tumor by a wide margin under age twenty-five. If you happen to be in that age bracket with a breast tumor, your doctor may give you reassurance that it's simply a benign tumor. His judgement is based on your age. He can not be sure by physical examination although in the face of a negative mammogram the diagnosis will probably be correct. After years of detecting these

Fig. 3-5
FIBROADENOMA. This lesion presents as a lump in the breast, usually in women under 30 years of age. The x-ray reveals a well demarcated white shadow in the upper part of the breast. The sharp border of the mass is characteristic of fibroadenoma. Nevertheless microscopic examination is mandatory to rule out cancer.

Fig. 3-6
BREAST BIOPSY OF FIBROADENOMA. Note the very sharp borders of this tumor. Fibroadenoma was confirmed on microscopic examination. The cause of fibroadenoma remains unknown.

lumps I must admit I've hazard a diagnosis like most surgeons. but I've always insisted that all such tumors be removed to definitely rule out cancer.

Some years ago a twenty-six year old black mother of two came to me for a second opinion about a lump in her breast. Yes, it was there, about as big as the end of your thumb. Freely movable, no pain. Mammogram showed the tumor. It appeared suspicious, but cancer was not definite.

"What'd your doctor tell you?", I asked.

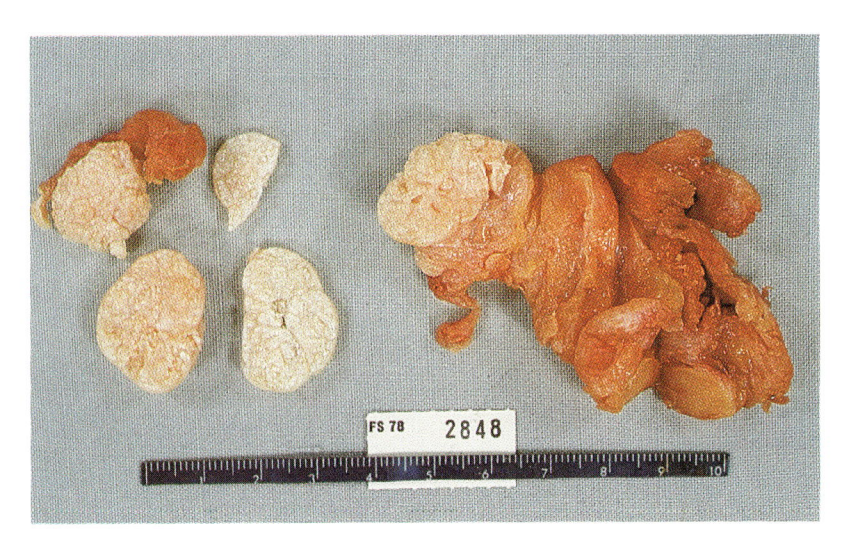

"Said it was a tumor, that was probably not a bad one, that I should have it out. What do you think, Doctor Johnson? I don't want to be experimented on if it's nothing to worry about."

"Well, I suppose your doctor wants it out just to be sure. Your mammogram was not diagnostic for cancer, even though there apparently was some irregularity. I agree that the chances are good that it is a benign tumor but we can't be completely sure unless we check it under the microscope. I'd have to agree with your doctor. Have it removed right away to be sure."

The young woman refused surgical removal of the lump. She wanted to wait and get another opinion. I saw her about a year or so later. She wanted me to check the lump. Sure enough the tumor was larger and seemed to be fixed to the underlying muscle. Enlarged lymph nodes were easily felt in the armpit.

She had **not** gotten another medical opinion afterall, and had only confided in friends. Now, there was pain. The growing tumor had been ignored as long as possible. Now she was forced to come to grips with the specter of cancer. Like so many other black women in our community she had allowed a malignancy to grow and spread. Only a few months later the cancer thief robbed another young family in spite of surgery, radiation and all the rest.

In real life Sherlock Holmes doesn't always win. The lesson to be learned is that regardless of your age, if a lump is felt in the breast do not delay seeking and accepting competent medical attention. Remember, only early cancer promptly treated is curable in more than 80 percent of cases.

SIFTING THE CLUES

Mammography (X-ray Examination)

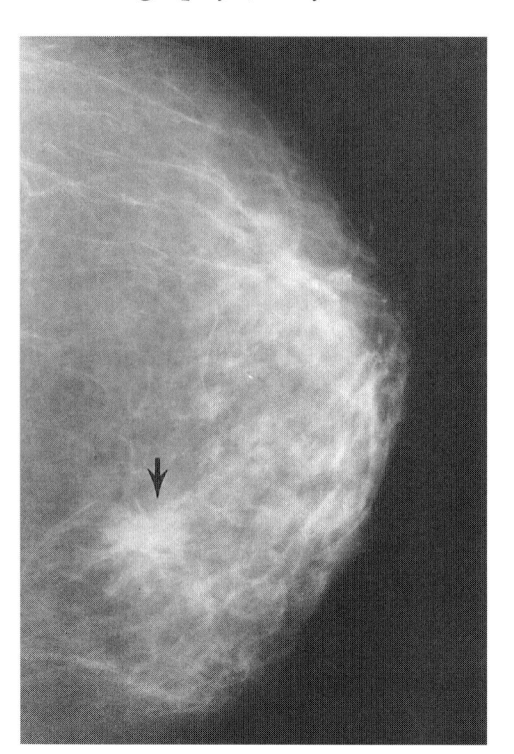

Along with BSE and periodic checks by the health provider, mammography (x-ray) examination of the breast has proven to be the most valuable tool for the medical detective.[10]

With the proliferation of

Fig. 3-7
MAMMOGRAMS. This mammogram reveals a suspicious area that demands biopsy. Today, x-rays of the breast are accomplished with extremely low radiation exposure. It is important that mammograms are performed at a facility that is approved by the American College of Radiology. Then you can be assured that the equipment is first rate, the technician is Registered, and the x-rays are being examined by a Board Certified Radiolgist. Mammograms are recommended beginning at age 40, according to the American Cancer Society.

> *Since black women show up with breast cancer seven years earlier than whites, I urge all black women to get their first baseline mammogram at age thirty.*
> • • • • • •

mammography screening centers it is important that the quality of the examinations be superior. If the center you choose is sanctioned by the American College of Radiology then you can be sure that it meets the highest standards and the report will be as accurate as possible.

In February, 1993 the feasibility of early mammography was raised. Data was presented at a National Cancer Institute conference that indicated that screening mammography before age 50 did not reduce breast cancer death rate in women ages 40 to 47.[21] Therefore some suggested that it was not cost effective to screen before age fifty. However, the American College of Radiology, the American Cancer Society, and other groups stated that the study was flawed and they continue to recommend screening every year from age forty. In my opinion, screening should begin at age 35 to make an impact on the 40 to 49 year old group. In fact I emphatically believe that all black women should be screened on a yearly basis from age 30, because the rate of cancer is one and a half times that of whites before age 35. Young black women are more likely to present with advanced disease, simply because it was not discovered in time. Screening mammography is still the best tool available.

Breast x-ray was first tried in the late 1940's. In those days machines were crude and radiation exposure was high. There was little enthusiasm for mammography early on and the technique lay fallow until the early 1960's, when investigators set about to improve mammography machines. Mammography first became available for a large population during a wide scale screening project sponsored by the New York Health Insurance Program, commonly called the HIP project. A modified x-ray machine had been developed that resulted in less radiation exposure and better defined negatives.[11]

Mammography continued to evolve along several pathways with improvement in the radiation producing apparatus and changes in the material upon which the image was recorded. In the early 1960's the French were developing an x-ray machine that used, instead of tungsten, molybdenum as a target for the x-rays. They also placed the anode closer to the target and found that these changes produced better definition in their images. In 1970 these alterations had been incorporated into a tidy efficient x-ray unit called the Senograph and marketed in the United States. It replaced the old tungsten x-ray model of the early 1960's. This new Senograph quite clearly detected very early cancers that could not be palpated.

Micro-calcifications and minute breast patterns indicative of malignancy were readily detected. There was also further reduction in radiation exposure with the new equipment from the seven to fifteen rads down to 2 $\frac{1}{2}$ rads.

About that time Dr John Wolfe reported on his experience in the development of xeroradiography (1968). The image was not recovered on a negative film as in the Senograph. It was imaged on a paper as a positive rendition. As a result, we now have two reliable and efficient methods widely available to uncover breast cancer before it can be palpated.

Nevertheless there was some question as to which was the better medium to view the mammogram, the celluloid film negative or the positive image on paper produced by the xeroradiograph. In the early days some technicians in training, and those at screening clinics preferred the xerograms. But many trained radiolgists accustomed to looking at negatives found

The radiation is now in the range of 0.2 to 0.3 rad, These are extremely low doses and the induction of breast cancer or other cancers by radiation is now of little or no significance.

that interpreting the negative film was satisfactory and in some cases preferable. In 1992 Xerox, the manufacturer of xeroradiograph paper announced that it would no longer produce that material since there was little demand for the product. The celluloid film is now the standard.

When hundreds and even thousands of women are being screened, use of the 105 mm roll Senograph film has definite advantages in being less expensive and requiring less time per patient. The Senograph film done on a long roll can be examined at the end of the screening day thus lessening time of the patient in the screening center, sometimes by as much as twenty minutes. On the other hand, the Xerox process allowed for little error in exposure and often repeat films were required.

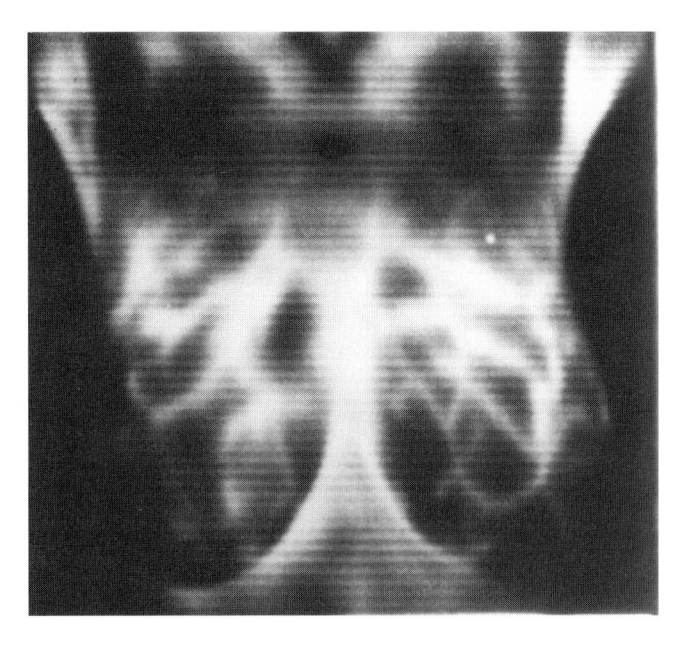

Fig. 3-8
NORMAL THERMOGRAPHY. Note the uniform dark areas in both breasts.

With improvement in film, screens, etc., the radiation exposure using the Senograph is now in the range of 0.2 to 0.3 rad, compared to 2 or 3 rads in xerograms. These are extremely low doses and the induction of breast cancer or other cancers by radiation is now of little or no significance. From various studies it has been estimated that using mammography of 0.3 rad there will result one extra case of breast cancer per million women screened after a ten year lag period. Even so, scientists are working on even more sophisticated equipment with xonics. This method will use electrons instead of photons to form the x-ray beam. They will produce images on Mylar instead of paper or celluloid and exposure will be reduced to only 0.05 to 0.1 rad.

Dr Wolfe found another use for mammography.[12] He theorized that cancer was very unlikely if certain patterns were found on the the mammogram. Other workers corroborated these findings. [13] The breast patterns reflecting a high density and cord structure and ductal hypertrophy developed cancer in 5 percent of the cases. The chance of developing cancer in a breast of low density and sparse ductless was only 0.5 percent. In either case the malignancy developed within three years. Other specialists, however, have remained skeptical and today, by and large, films with differing patterns are not used to predict the chance of cancer development.

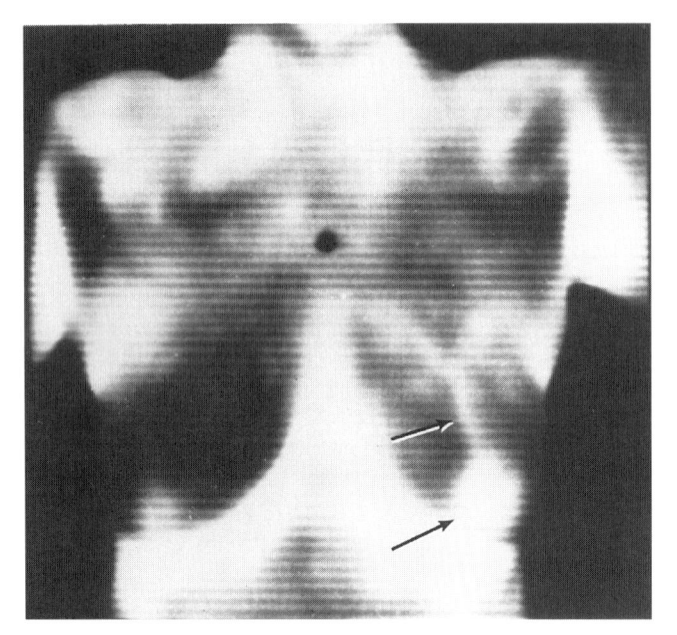

Thermography

The tools of the medical Sherlock Holmes do not stop with mammography and its various developments. Also available is thermography [14]. There is some controversy regarding its usefulness, although some physicians find it helpful. This device is a heat sensor apparatus that is designed to record differences in temperature throughout the breast onto a permanent record. Malignant breast lesions often have a higher temperature than normal breast tissue and some success has been noted in detecting early cancer that was otherwise obscure. Inflammatory disease and benign tumors can also register an increased temperature; and the method has been found to be fraught with frequent false negative and false positive findings. Consequently most

Fig. 3-9
ABNORMAL THERMOGRAPHY. Note the white shadow (arrow) in the left breast that is highly suspicious of cancer. Thermography is not as good as mammography when screening for breast cancer; but it may be useful to confirm a suspicious lesion that will prompt your doctor to recommend a biopsy.

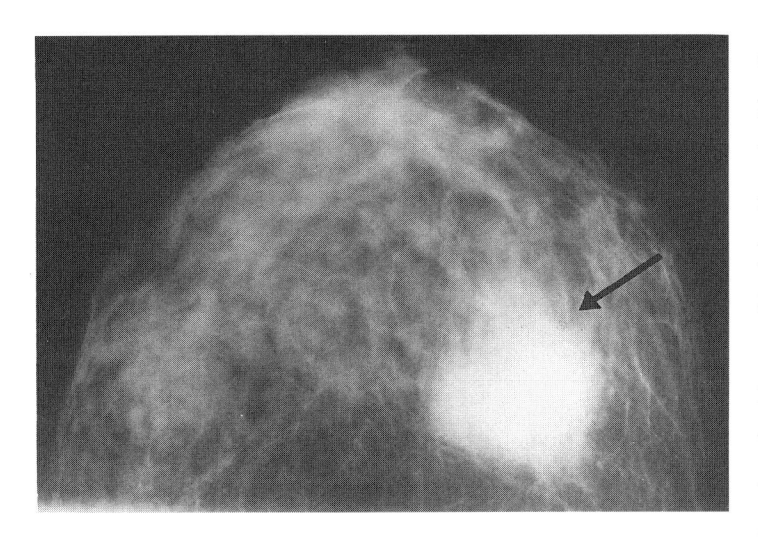

Fig. 3-10
BREAST MASS. IS IT SOLID OR FILLED WITH FLUID? If the x-ray reveals a large mass, it may well be a harbinger of cancer. However if it is a cyst it can be drained and the mass will disappear.

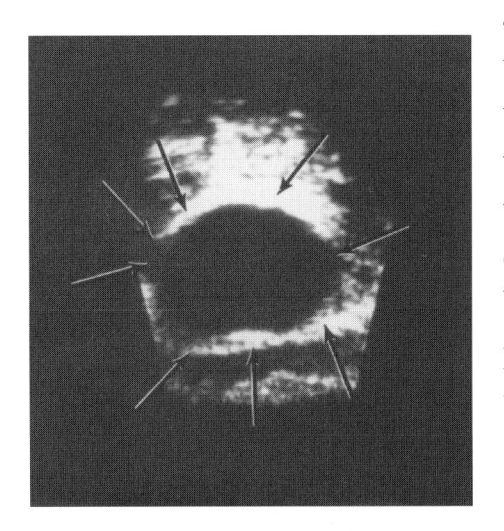

Fig. 3-11
ULTRASOUND. By using the ultrasound it can be determined if a mass is solid and possibly a cancer or simply a fluid filled cyst. In this case the ultrasound showed only a fluid-filled cyst that was drained. The fluid was examined for cancer cells; none were found and the cyst did not return.

centers do not rely on thermography for anything more than a confirmatory technique in the face of positive physical and/or mammographic findings.

Some screening centers noting a 20 percent false positive rate have omitted the thermography altogether. Others still argue that thermography is of some benefit in the doubtful case. Occasional so-called false positive cases do indeed develop a breast cancer two to three years later. If the mammogram is equivocal and the physical examination is not definite then a positive thermogram would be likely to prompt breast biopsy.

I have never personally ordered a thermography study for my patients. I just don't feel that the expense is justified. If a lump is suspicious on the mammogram a biopsy must be done regardless of the results from the thermogram.

Thermography is defined by the American College of Radiology and American Thermographic Society as a "complimentary diagnostic tool" that may be useful in the evaluation of breast disease when combined with both physical examination and mammography under the supervision of a

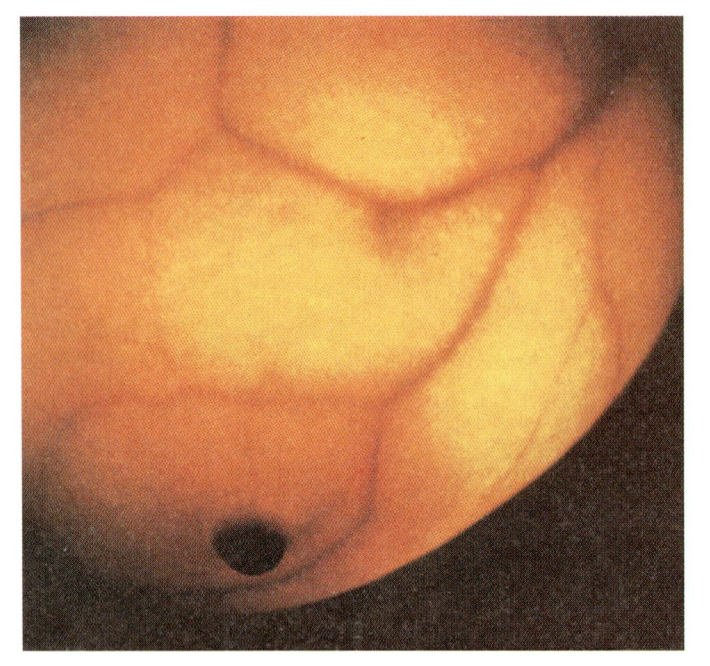

Fig. 3-12
NORMAL DIAPHANOGRAM. The color is a uniform yellow color on transillumination which depicts a normal breast.

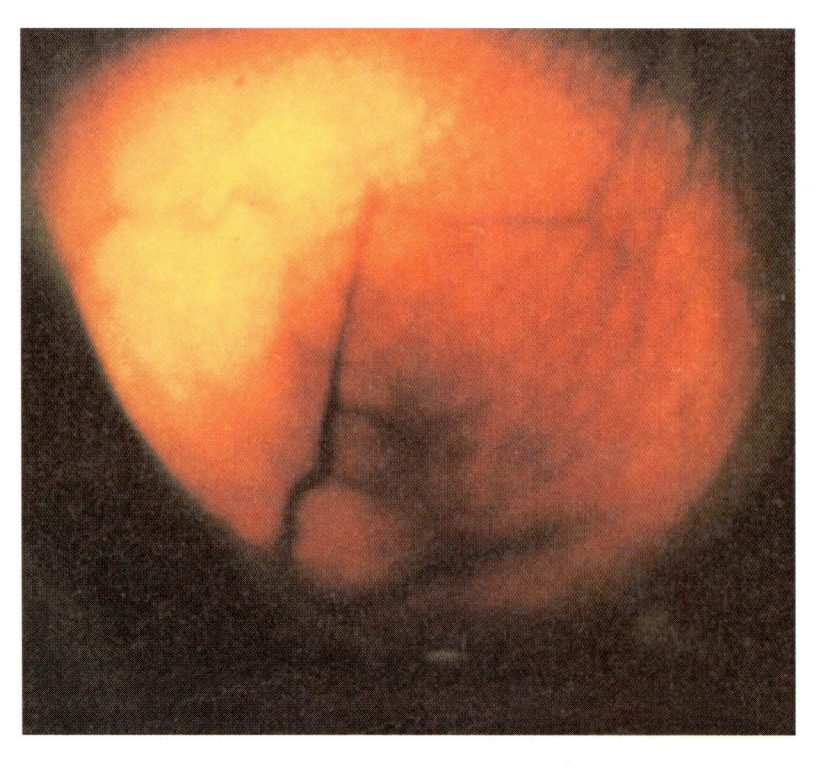

Fig. 3-13
ABNORMAL DIAPHANOGRAM. Note the dark irregular shadow in the lower right portion of the breast. This is highly suggestive of cancer. This test is seldom done today because the accuracy does not nearly approach mammography.

qualified physician and a trained radiologist.

Ultrasound

The ultrasound machine is a device that uses sound waves to distinguish solid masses from cysts. It operates on the principle that the density of cystic and solid structures reflect sound waves differently and thereby produce images that are easily differentiated. The accuracy in detecting cancer is only 60 to 75 percent. It finds its greatest usefulness in examining young women with dense breast tissue when a cyst is suspected.[15]

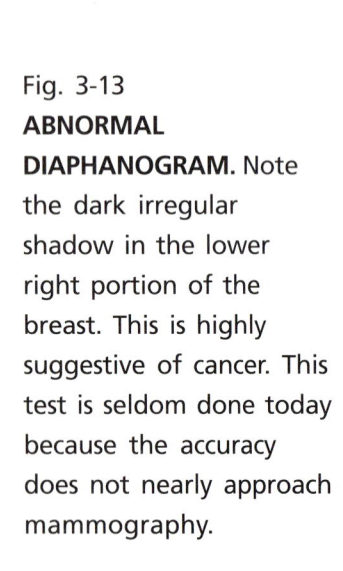

Many surgeons, including myself, rely heavily on ultrasound to distinguish cystic and solid masses. It's a good idea to always get an ultrasound study before needle aspiration of a breast lump.

Diaphanography

This is a fairly recent addition to the family of breast imaging techniques. It does not replace x-ray mammography, but may uncover very early cancers not detected by the mammogram. This is not a certainty, however, and its usefulness is still being evaluated. Presently, its principle use is to confirm what is found by other detecting methods. It involves transillumination with infrared and photographing the result. The picture is then carefully examined for defects.[16]

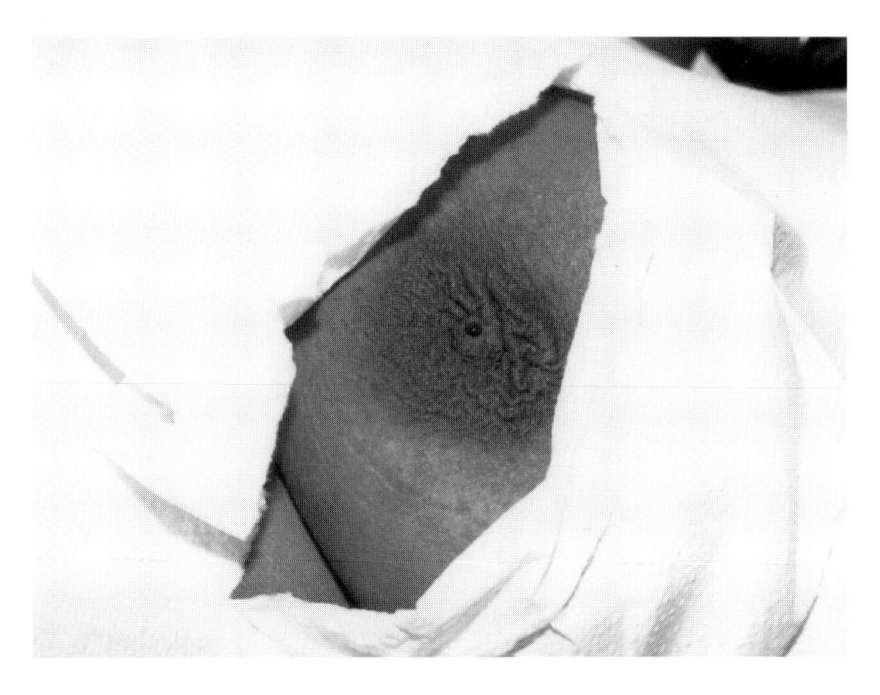

Nipple discharge

Fluid discharging spontaneously from the nipple or provoked by gentle pressure may be either cloudy or blood tinged. The question of cancer, of course, is uppermost on the mind if one experiences blood or any fluid coming from the breast. In the majority of cases a benign lesion (papilloma) is the cause, but cancer is found with increasing frequency in older age groups.

Breast cancers are associated with a bloody fluid discharge about 20 percent of the time even though a lump is not readily palpable. Therefore careful detec-

Fig. 3-14
BLOOD COMING FROM NIPPLE. Breast cancers are associated with a bloody fluid discharge about 20 percent of the time even though a lump is not readily palpable.

tive work will mandate an x-ray exam and probably biopsy in the case of bloody discharge from the nipple.

On the other hand, a thin clear fluid discharge may be noted for years and be completely benign. If the discharge is copious and clear it may signal the presence of a a prolactinoma tumor of the pituitary.

Biopsy

Whenever a mass or lump is located by palpation and/or mammo-graphy, etc., the next step is to obtain tissue for absolute identification. In many clinics the breast biopsy is done on an out-patient basis under local anesthesia. however if the breast is pendulous or the lesion small and difficult to locate the surgeon may elect to hospitalize the patient and do the biopsy under general anesthesia with preliminary needle localization.

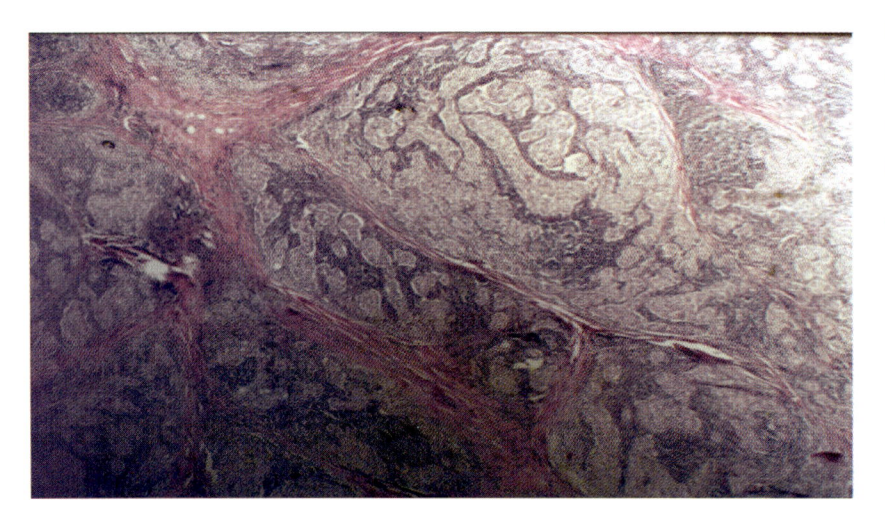

Fig. 3-15
BREAST CANCER UNDER THE MICROSCOPE
The gray-purple cells are cancer.

Many physicians prefer not to perform a mastectomy at the time of biopsy if the specimen is found to be cancerous. On the other hand some patients prefer immediate mastectomy if the biopsy is positive. I encourage postponing mastectomy following biopsy so that the tissue removed can be examined in greater detail after it is properly fixed and stained. That takes about two days. In the meantime the patient and family can discuss the ramifications of various treatment options. It is not unusual for a patient to decide in favor of another treatment option even though mastectomy was the initial decision. So a short delay may be wise. According to a study done by Dr Fisher and his group, there is absolutely no adverse affect if mastectomy is delayed for two weeks after the biopsy.[17]

Before submitting to the standard biopsy, you may wish to discuss the possibility of aspiration cytology or core needle biopsy. In many centers these biopsy methods are being used more frequently. Needle aspiration has almost no complications and is much less discomforting than open biopsy.

Before submitting to the standard biopsy, you may wish to discuss the possibility of needle biopsy.

Chest X-ray

The chest x-ray is one of the first clues to be examined in all cases of suspected breast cancer. Metastasis to the lung can be detected and if a solitary lesion found, surgical excision may be possible. If many lesions are present then proper chemotherapy or radiation should be used.

Bone Scan and Liver Scan

The bone scan is seldom done in the early and mid-stages of breast cancer. Unless there is bone pain or specific complaints the chance of finding a bone metastasis is less than 21 percent. On the other hand liver scan is worthwhile early on. It should be preceded by a much less expensive blood test. If the blood test is positive for some unidentified liver problem then the scan may be of assistance in diagnosing cancer.

Blood Tests

The alkaline phosphatase blood determination becomes elevated early in liver metastasis. Anywhere from 60-90 percent of those with breast cancer and liver spread will have an elevated result. All blood tests have limited value. The alkaline phosphatase can also be abnormal in a number of other unrelated conditions. A blood test to detect only cancer is not presently available. Of course it would be the ideal screening device and investigators are struggling to bring it into reality. Indeed, such a discovery would all but eliminate our prolonged detective endeavors.

Another important blood test requiring careful interpretation is the Carcino-embryonic Antigen (CEA).[18] This substance is elevated in about 50 percent of breast cancer patients. It is also observed in the blood of some patients with colon cancer and cancer of the pancreas. CEA may also be elevated in the case of liver cirrhosis, emphysema, peptic ulcer, and colitis. Nevertheless the CEA blood level should be checked if breast cancer is suspected. If cancer is later confirmed and adequately treated the CEA blood level should fall to normal in most cases. Any subsequent rise in the CEA may herald a recurrence of the malignancy even if there are no other clues. It has been noted that if the CEA level falls below 2.5 nanagrams following treatment (surgery or radiation) there is a 20 percent chance of recurrence in the ensuing two year period. If the CEA fails to fall below that point the recurrence rate is 65 percent during the following two year post-treatment period.[19]

A new test, the DNA histogram is useful in predicting whether a cancer will be aggressive leading to early recurrence and a poor prognosis.[20]

―――

In all of these careful investigations to uncover the breast cancer perpetrator, the physician must be knowledgable and persistent just like Holmes the detective. The investigation must be organized in a logical and straight-forward manner leading to the diagnosis. This can only be achieved successfully with the support and cooperation of the patient herself.

It is true, we cannot predict who will contract breast cancer. At the same time all of us must be just as aware as Sherlock Holmes and other good detectives, of various premonitory conditions. In the next chapter you will have an opportunity to examine those risk factors as I attempt to answer the question: 'Who Gets Breast Cancer?'

REFERENCES

1. Strax P: Advances in detection of early breast cancer; Cancer detection and prevention. 6:409-414 1983 pub. Alan R Liss Inc

2. Young JL, Devesa SS, Cutler SJ: Incidence of cancer in United States Blacks. Cancer Research 35:3523-3536 Nov 1975

3. Foster RS, Costanza MC: Breast self-examination practices and breast cancer survival. Cancer 53:4 999-1005 Feb 15 1984

4. Lesnick GL: How best to proceed when the diagnosis is 'fibrocystic breast disease'. Your Patient and Cancer Feb 1983

5. Greenblatt RB, Nexhat C, Ben-Hur J: Treatment of benign breast disease with danazol. Fertil Steril 34:242 1980

6. Goldenburg IS, Gump FE, Minton JP, et al: When breasts are fibrocystic. Patient Care 16:103-107 March 1982

7. Black MM, Barclay THC, Cutler SJ, Hankey BF, et al: Association of atypical characteristics of benign breast lesions with subsequent risk of breast cancer. Cancer 29:338-343 1972

8. Devitt JE: Breast cancer and preceding clinical benign breast disorders-a chance association. Lancet 793-795 April 10, 1976

9. Groveman HD, Norcross WA: Adolescent breast masses. Hospital Medicine 65-84 May 1982

10. Lester RG: Risk versus benefit in mammography. Radiology 124:1 1977

11. Shapiro S, Strax P, Venet L: Periodic breast cancer screening in reducing mortality from breast cancer. JAMA 215: 1777-1785 1971

12. Wolf JN: Risk for breast cancer development determined by mammographic parenchymal pattern. Cancer 37:2486 1976

13. Krook PM, Carlile T, Bush W, et al: Mammographic parenchymal patterns as a risk indicator for prevalent and incident cancer. Cancer 41:1093-1097 1978

14. Gautherie M, Gross CM: Breast thermography and cancer risk prediction. Cancer 45:51-56 Jan 1980

15. Teixidor HS, Elias K: Combined mammographic-sonographic evaluation of the breast. March 1977

16. Toomes H, Vogt-Moykopf I: Surgery advised for palli-

ative treatment of lung metastases. Reported at 14th annual Congress on Diseases of the Chest (American College of Chest Physicians). Family Practice News 13:3 Feb 1-14 1983 pp 85

17. Fisher E Sass R Fisher B :Biological considerations regarding the one and two step procedures in the management of patients with invasive carciinoma of the breast. SG&O 161:245-249 September 1985

18. Lee, YTW, CEA in patients with breast...cancer, West J Med 129:374-380 Nov 1978

19. Tormey DC Waalkes TP Snyder JJ Simon RM :Biological markers in breast carcinoma. III. Clinical correlations with carcinoembryonic antigen. Cancer 1977 Jun;(6) :2397-2404

20. Olszewski W Zbigniew D Rosen PP et al :Flow Cytometry of breast carcinoma: I. Relation of DNA Plody Level to histology and estrogen receptor. Cancer 48:4 Aug 15 1981 980-988

21. "Value of mammograms in younger women questioned": Amer Med News page 3; March 22/29 1993

Incentive for mammography are (1) a doctor's recommendation, (2) personal experience from family or a friend, and (3) information from the media. The doctor's recommendation is far and away the strongest incentive. Therefore all doctors must take a particular responsibility to alert women of this danger.

Glockner SM, Hilton SVW, Holden MG, et al; Women's attitude towards screening mammography: American Journal of Preventive Medicine 8:69-77, 1992

CHAPTER FOUR

THE FICKLE FINGER OF FATE
Who Gets Breast Cancer?

*t*he incidence of **lung cancer** among women is gaining with 46,000 new cases in 1985 and over 50,000 new cases found in 1989; and the rate is expected to increase into the 1990's. but those numbers are not even close to the epidemic of breast cancer.

Today, one out of every eight American women, black and white, will contract breast cancer. In 1975 70,000 new cases were discovered. In 1981 109,000 cases were found. By 1985 119,000 new cases were added. Then in 1989 we saw 143,000 new breast cancer patients. In 1990 the figure rose to over 150,000 and in 1991 **175,000** new cases were reported. The American Cancer Society estimates that **183,000** new cases will be found in the United States in 1993.[38] There can be no doubt: **This is by far the number one cancer facing *all* women in the United States.**

Now let's look at some figures according to race. The National Cancer Institute reported that breast cancer in 1973 was diagnosed in 65.6 black women and 82.9 white women per hundred thousand population. By 1981 the number of black women with breast cancer had increased by 12 percent to 75 per hundred thousand while the incidence among whites

*The American Cancer Society estimates that **183,000** new cases will be found in the United States in 1993.*
● ● ● ● ● ● ● ●

had increased only six percent.[1]

Other government studies emphasize the marked difference in the occurrence of breast cancer and mortality between black and white women.[2] Mortality among black women is 10 percent higher than whites.[42] The figures point up the likelihood that black women are contracting breast cancer so fast that by the year 2000 the relative number will surpass the occurrence among white women and the mortality will continue to be higher.

The problem of breast cancer is particularly acute among young black women when you consider the prevalence of cancer before the age of 40. An early study showed that from age 35 to 39 the incidence of breast cancer is 69.5 among blacks, compared to 59.0 for whites per hundred thousand population.[1] A recent study revealed that before age 35 the incidence of breast cancer among black women is one and a half times the rate of white women.[41]

There is little wonder that women of all stations—rich and poor, black and white—are at least concerned if not downright alarmed.

I remember a young black woman timidly raising her hand during a question-answer period following one of my presentations. After she was recognized, she stood and in a small voice asked, 'How will I know if I'm likely to get breast cancer, other than being a woman? I mean is there any thing that makes me more apt to get cancer than the next woman. You know what I mean? Is it just luck or something? You know what I mean?'

The young woman was asking, in her own way, 'What are the risk factors for getting breast cancer? What can we look for and prepare for, or is it just the fickle finger of fate?'

"For most women there are no over-riding risk factors that we know of. In fact researchers have shown that there are no known risk factors in 70 percent of breast cancer cases. On the other hand there are risk factors in 20 percent of younger women and in about 30 percent of older women."[38]

So in this chapter I will review those markers that we know may increase your likelihood of acquiring breast cancer.

RISK FACTORS FOR BREAST CANCER

Advancing Age

In Europe and in the United States breast cancer rates are directly proportional to advancing age. American women, black and white, at age 60 are more prone to cancer than those at age 40, and age 70 bears an increased risk over the woman at age sixty. There is a 30 fold increase in breast cancer risk from age 25 to 65.[3,4]

Heredity

It has long been recognized that some breast cancer patients, both black and white, are clustered in families such as sisters, mother and sister(s), mother and daughter and other combinations.[5]

Before the menopause these breast cancers with family ties are more often found than cancers that occur after the change of life. Hence, the premenopausal woman whose mother had breast cancer before her change of life will have a three fold increased chance of also developing breast cancer. A woman with a mother who had breast cancer after her menopause will have only a 1.2 increased risk of breast

A recent study revealed that before age 35 the incidence of breast cancer among black women is one and a half times the rate of white women.

cancer. Investigators at the M.D Anderson Hospital in Houston examined the relatives of postmenopausal cancer patients who had cancer in both breasts. They found that close relatives had a four fold increase in breast cancer. Close relative of premenopausal women who had cancer in both breasts had a nine-fold increased risk of breast cancer.[5]

Without taking menopause into account, statistics show that a woman in the United States, with a sister or mother with breast cancer, carries a life-time risk of one in five of contracting breast cancer. If the sister and mother both had breast cancer then the woman's chances of getting breast cancer increased to one chance in two life-time risk. Her breast cancer would most likely strike before age 40 and would often be in both breasts.[6] As mentioned earlier, genetic factors seem to affect risk more often before menopause when ovarian estrogen plays a major role. Probably environmental factors take over the causative role in later life.[5]

Female sex vs. Male sex

It is true that females have an overwhelming number of breast cancers compared to males. Consequently, the female sex, per se, is a risk factor. The National Cancer Institute reported that in the five year period 1973 through 1977 only 40 breast cancers were found in black males compared to 3,118 in black females.[2] It's not surprising that many physicians complete their entire medical careers without seeing a single case of **male** breast cancer. The rates are 72 black females per hundred thousand compared to 1.4 black males per hundred thousand. The concern is that a man may harbor a breast lump, suspecting some benign misfortune when a cancer is actually growing and spreading. As a result, studies reveal,

> **M**any physicians complete their entire medical careers without seeing a single case of **male** breast cancer.
> • • • • • • •

most breast cancers in the male are large and have metastasized when finally diagnosed. The mortality is correspondingly high, simply because this rare male cancer was never suspected in its early stage.

Injury

Some women report a lump in the breast after a minor injury that draws their attention, leading them to carefully palpate the breast. If the lump they discover subsequently proves to be cancerous, the inference follows that the injury may have caused the cancer. As far as I can tell, there are no studies that demonstrate a causal link between injury and cancer of the breast. The injury caused by chapped and cracking nipples seen in the nursing breast and in non-pregnant women can cause infection; but, apparently, it does not lead to cancer. However, a bruise can lead to a lump of fat necrosis which may be indistinguishable from breast cancer even on mammogram and will thus require biopsy.

Parity

This refers to the number of children a woman has birthed. Having a child at age twenty or younger decreases the chance of breast cancer significantly and having a child before age thirty also confers some protection. After the first child there is no further protection in having more children.[7] A woman who is nulliparous, that is, who's never carried a child to full term is at greater risk for breast cancer. On the other hand, a first child born after age 35 triples the risk of breast cancer.[8]

Breast Feeding

Studies have failed to show a consistent relationship between breast feeding (Figure 4-1) or the lack of breast feeding and the subsequent development of breast cancer. One investigation from Japan (a low risk country) suggested there was some protection in prolonged breast feeding where lactation up to 5 to 10 years occurred frequently.[8] A review of the world-wide literature would indicate that prolonged nursing probably has little if any effect on the incidence of breast cancer.

Radiation

There is no doubt that radiation can cause breast cancer.[9] In fact radiation exposure can increase the incidence of cancer 2 to 3 times. That is why chest x-rays must be kept to a minimum and the dosage of mammography carefully controlled. A study reported in 1965 revealed that women who received multiple fluoroscopic examinations had a high incidence of breast cancer over a ten year period.[10] It was also shown that the cancer developed on the side of the chest that received the radiation.

Other data examined Japanese women exposed to the radiation from the atomic blasts over Hiroshima and Nagasaki.[11] After observing this group for ten years the investigators concluded that women exposed to 90 rads or more of radiation would develop

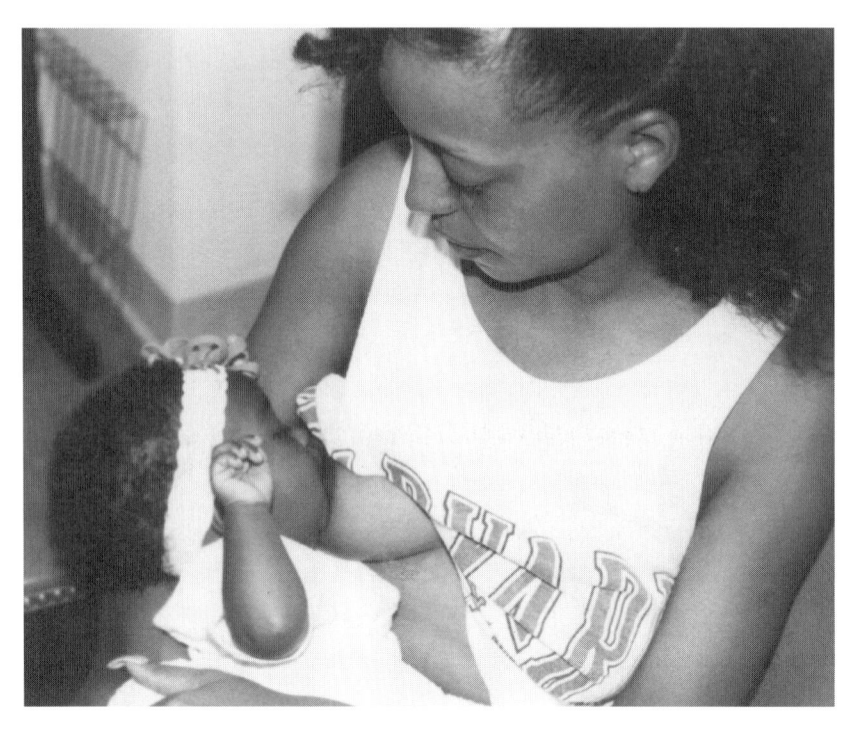

Fig. 4-1
Breast Feeding does not seem to have a bearing on the development of Breast Cancer. Nor does it protect against the occurrence of breast cancer.

breast cancer at a rate two to four times that of an otherwise comparable population.

Fibrocystic Dysplasia

There seems to be a definite relationship between fibrocystic dysplasia (Figure 4-2) and breast cancer. Although the mechanism remains unclear, several reports agree that women with fibrocystic dysplasia develop cancer four times as often as otherwise normal women.[12,13]

Breast cancer and fibro-cystic dysplasia, it is believed, are induced by estrogen, the hormone produced by the ovary. The reason that some women respond to this hormone and develop benign fibrocystic dysplasia and others go on to malignant breast cancer is unknown. In some cases fibrocystic dysplasia forms so many dense nodules in the breasts it may be impossible to distinguish a cancer by palpation alone. Mammography may be useful although many times biopsy of a suspicious nodule is required for proper diagnosis.

More recent reports indicate fibrocystic dysplasia and other benign breast diseases represent a marker for possible development of cancer if there is atypia or cell abnormalities found in the biopsy specimen. However, even without atypia, there is a modest increased incidence of cancer developing.[40]

Lobular Carcinoma In Situ

This is one of the clearest markers of the possibility

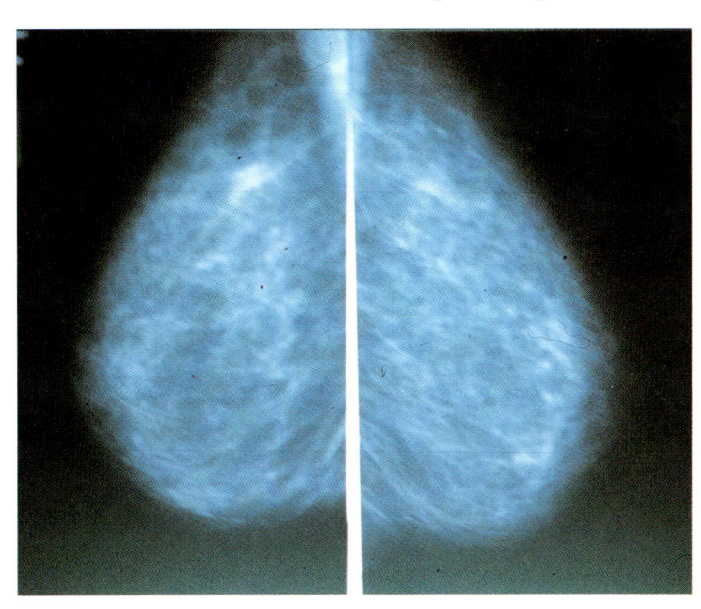

Fig. 4-2
Fibrocystic Dysplasia. This mammogram is similar to the fibrocystic dysplasia shown in Chapter 3.
The mammogram shows multiple round dark shadows that are firm nodules throughout both breasts. These lumps may hide a cancer and in some cases your doctor may reccommend repeating the mammogram in six months. Of course, biopsy is mandatory in suspicious cases.

Cancer in one breast predisposes a woman to cancer in the opposite breast.
• • • • • • •

of cancer developing in a breast. In the past several years with the increased use of mammography this lesion is found more and more. It cannot be felt by simple palpation. It usually appears as a cluster of calcium grains on a routine mammogram. When LCIS is confirmed at biopsy, one can be sure that in 20 to 30 percent of cases a cancer will develop in **either** breast. This requires very careful mammograms yearly or more frequently. Some patients, particularly with a strong family history of breast cancer opt for bilateral mastectomy rather than take the risk. This may be a drastic option since you find the incidence increasing only one percent per year for the first ten years.

Cancers associated with Breast Cancer

Cancer in one breast predisposes a woman to cancer in the opposite breast, and thus, presents a risk factor. Ten percent of breast cancer patients will develop cancer in the opposite breast, and depending on the cellular type, the rate may be higher.[5] Indeed, it has been reported that a biopsy of the normal breast in the spot that cancer was found in the cancerous breast revealed hidden cancer in the 'normal' breast in 20 percent of cases.

There is a direct relation between **cancer of the uterus** and breast cancer. Apparently, estrogen or other unknown factors that lead to malignant degeneration of the uterine lining are also associated with breast malignancy. This combination occurs twice as often as noted in the general population. Hence, in every patient with proven cancer of the uterus, careful surveillance for breast cancer is mandatory and vice-versa.

Cancer of the ovary and breast cancer also arise

together more often than expected by chance alone, but the connection is more tenuous than the breast cancer-uterine cancer combination.

Ovarian cancer and uterine cancer are also found together for unknown reasons. A common stimulus is suspected since these cancer combinations, when they do occur, are found within a few years of one another.

Even more mysterious and fickle is the association of breast cancer and **colon cancer.** Some workers have shown that breast cancer follows the discovery of colon cancer more often than expected. So colon cancer is considered a risk factor. Populations at risk for colon malignancies, primarily Europeans and those ascribing to the diet of western cultures, consume a high fat content in their foods and this leads to a bacterial flora in the intestines which produces steroid compounds and estrogens which may be carcinogenic (able to cause cancer) for both colon and breast.

Finally, there is some association between breast cancer and **leukemia**; and cancer of the **salivary glands** increases the likelihood of breast cancer by four in both black and white women.

Female Hormones produced in the body and Breast Cancer

We know that the hormone estrogen produced in the ovary is responsible for the female persona: the smooth hairless face, the rounded contoured physiognomy, the development of breast tissue, and menstruation. In Chapter Two it was pointed out that the onset of menstruation signals a sharply increased flow of estrogen from the developing ovaries; and we know that the longer a woman is exposed to estrogen the

Women whose first pregnancy was before age 20 had only one-half the breast cancer risk as women whose first pregnancy was after age 25.

• • • • • • •

greater the chance of contracting breast cancer. Investigators have confirmed that females who begin menstruating early, perhaps at age nine or ten, and women who have a late menopause at age fifty-five instead of forty-five, will have an increased risk of cancer simply because they were exposed to estrogen a few years longer.

Conversely, women that have had their ovaries removed by surgery before the menopause have less breast cancer because of the shorter exposure time to estrogen. Males produce only minute amounts of estrogen, and develop breast cancer at a rate less than one percent of that found in the female. In experimental animals such as mice, hamsters and rabbits, breast cancer can be produced without fail by the injection of estrogen. All of these facts point to the central role of estrogen in producing human breast cancer.

Looking further, we find that there are actually three types of estrogen produced by the ovary: Estrone, Estradiol, and Estriol. This is absolutely important to understand since only the estrone and estradiol fractions are carcinogenic. Estrone and estradiol regularly produce breast cancer in the laboratory animal.

Estriol, however, not only fails to cause cancer, it can inhibit the estrone and estradiol estrogens.[14]

Ovaries of black Africans, Orientals and other non-whites produce mostly estriol. In Caucasians, the estrone and estradiol fractions are the predominant hormones. This is an accepted fact. The high rates of breast cancer in whites compared to the rarity in black Africans and Orientals corresponds to the prevalence of estrone and estradiol in Caucasians and the predominance of estriol in non-whites. This finding was confirmed when cmparing the estrogens of black Africans, whites and Indians in Zambia. Another study compared the estrogen types in Japanese women to those of a white population. The ovaries of white women produce these estrogen fractions more than any other race and they produce the vast majority of breast cancer the world over.[15]

During pregnancy, the ovaries of all women, both black and white begin to elaborate large quantities of estriol, the safe estrogen. If pregnancy takes place before age nineteen, this surge of estriol will give a measure of protection against any breast cancer that would have occurred before age forty-five.

As a matter of fact, a study from Brazil in 1971 demonstrated that women whose first pregnancy was before age 20 had only one-half the breast cancer risk as women whose first pregnancy was after age 25.[16]

Dr Henry M. Lemon at the University of Nebraska has shown quite dramatically that estriol can prevent estrone and estradiol from causing breast cancer in animals.[14]

Ten years later Dr Lemon described the high incidence of estrone and estradiol in breast cancer patients and he wondered aloud if we shouldn't give estriol (the anti-cancer estrogen) to help prevent cancer in women who have low levels of this hormone.[17] Clearly this question can only be addressed when The Food and Drug Administration allows clinical trials to proceed.

Someone asked, "If breast cancer is caused by female hormones, why does cancer continue to rise in the elderly after the ovaries stop producing hormones?"

No one has the complete answer, although there are credible theories. With the menopause or change

> *Women who have a late menopause at age fifty-five instead of forty-five, will have an increased risk of cancer simply because they were exposed to estrogen a few years longer.*

of life, the estrogen level drops off as the ovaries begin to involute and atrophy. At that point the fickle finger beckons the adrenal and pituitary glands to take over and produce hormones that can be just as provocative in the development of breast cancer.

The adrenals, one small gland located above each kidney, manufacture a host of hormones, many of which are absolutely essential to life. They also produce some non-essential hormones including androstenidione and our old friend estrone, which, you will recall, is one of the cancer causing estrogens.

Only 2 percent of the estrone is produced directly by the adrenals[18], Ninety eight percent is produced indirectly by way of the androstenidione.

After the menopause, androstenidione, from the adrenal glands, has the capacity and does indeed produce estrone from the body's fat cells; and the more fat depots present the more estrone can be manufactured, and consequently, the greater potential for breast cancer.

It should be noted that androstenidione also induces the pituitary gland, located on the under surface of the brain, to secrete prolactin.

Prolactin, produced by the pituitary gland in the brain, is a hormone that is absolutely necessary for the production of breast milk. It also promotes cancer in the presence of estrone. Some patients with breast cancer have high blood levels of prolactin. In fact close family members of some breast cancer patients have elevated prolactin levels. This may serve as a marker of relatives (mother, daughter, sister) that require special observation for cancer development.[18,19]

Hypophysectomy (surgical removal of the pituitary gland) has been an effective paliative treatment of metastatic breast cancer, probably due to the elimination of prolactin. Effective drugs that will bring consistent and sustained lowering of prolactin levels are being tested. Thus far, no drug that lowers prolactin level has proven to be satisfactory for breast cancer control.

The chemical dimethylbenzanthracene (DMBA) is used experimentally to induce breast cancer in mice. If the animal is placed on high fat rations, cancer is produced much faster and more consistently.[4]

Prescribed Hormones for Hot Flashes and Breast Cancer

For more than fifty years American women have been spared the nuisance and sometimes anguish of the menopause through the judicious use of hormones. These hormones, of course, are estrogens or estrogen-like medications. They have an excellent record of controlling the hot flashes, insomnia, perspiration, and anxiety that are sometimes a part of the change of life. In view of the carcinogenic consequences produced in the laboratory animal, a woman should be concerned about the propensity of these pills to cause human cancer.

A study from the Harvard School of Public Health is instructive. These investigators followed 1,891 menopausal women who were taking estrogens to alleviate hot flashes.[20] These women were matched against the general population of the same age that were not taking hormone. The groups were then observed over a fifteen year period. For the first ten years there was no difference in the rate of breast cancer. After 12 years, it was noted that there was a 30 percent increased rate of breast cancer in those taking high doses of hormone for hot flashes.

After 15 years of surveillance, women on high doses of estrogens showed twice the amount of breast can-

> *After 15 years of surveillance, women on high doses of estrogens showed twice the amount of breast cancer as the control.*

cer as the control. Low dose patients did not have a significant increment of breast cancer. This study also showed that breast cancer was higher in women that used estrogens three weeks out of the month rather than continuously. If fibrocystic dysplasia was present prior to using estrogens for menopausal symptoms, breast cancer occurred twice as often as the general population. If fibrocystic disease became evident following the use of these hormones, the fickle finger of cancer struck seven times more often then in the general population.[21]

Birth Control Pills and Breast Cancer

Medication produced for contraception generally contain an estradiol and an estrone-like hormone. Some also contain progesterone. The hormones in these medications are kept very low to avoid side effects. Women with known risk factors for breast cancer are cautioned to be extra vigilant. Package inserts clearly warn of the danger of birth control pills combined with such risk factors as fibrocystic dysplasia, prior history of breast cancer, or family history of breast cancer.

A study on the subject published in 1975 showed that women, black and white, who used oral contraception for two to four years increased their chances of contracting breast cancer two and a half times. Usage of less than two years or more than four years was not associated with increased risk. However, if benign fibrocystic disease was present and proven with biopsy then long-term use of birth control medication (six or more years) lead to an eleven fold increase of breast cancer.[21]

A more recent analysis by the Centers for Disease Control in 1982 suggested that oral contraceptives do

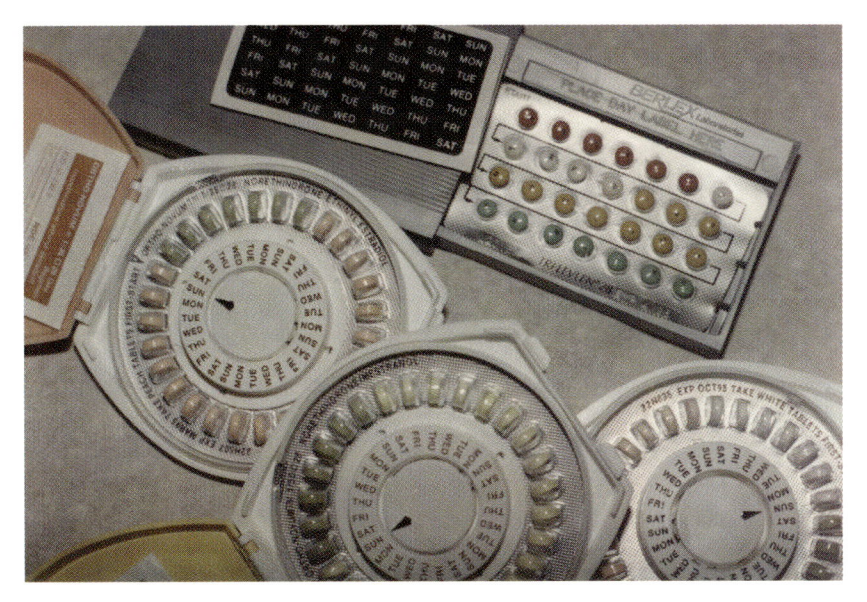

Fig. 4-3
Birth Control Pills may or may not increase the incidence of breast cancer. There are conflicting reports. The insert that comes with all birth control pills warns against use if there are any known risk factors present.

not increase the risk of breast cancer. In fact their observations indicate that there is probably a beneficial effect in reducing the likelihood of contracting endometrial cancer (cancer of the womb).[22]

The New York State Cancer Control Bureau reported in 1983 that there was an increased risk of breast cancer in women on birth control pills whose grandmothers had breast cancer. Their data also suggested that there was no increased risk if sister or mother had had cancer. Further, breast cancer risk was decreased among birth control users if there was no family history of breast cancer.

Much of the literature from Europe would link the use of oral contraceptives to breast cancer. Occasional articles in American journals also raise the association of breast cancer and birth control pills.[39-42]

All of this conflicting information gives you some idea of the differing experiences being reported, and the likelihood of confusion. My advice is to go along with the package insert and avoid birth control pills if there are other risk factors present. If there are no other contraindications, then oral contraceptives represent a viable option for birth control. Nevertheless there is enough data to warrant caution.

Thyroid and Breast Cancer

The thyroid gland is an "H" shaped gland found in

the neck. It produces thyroxine and other hormones that control the body metabolism. When the gland is overactive it sometimes enlarges forming a goiter and causes the heart to beat fast, the nerves to become tremulous, and weight loss in spite of a ravishing appetite. If the gland is underactive the body becomes sluggish and overweight.

One becomes cold easily, the hair thins and face and hands become puffy.

In the postmenopausal years women are prone to have an underactive thyroid and are often placed on thyroid supplement medication. A report appearing in the Journal of the American Medical Association in 1976 analyzed 635 patients who were receiving thyroid medication and compared them with 4,870 women not on thyroid medication. These populations were followed for fifteen years. Women on thyroid supplement had twice the rate of breast cancer as women not on thyroid medication. When the group on thyroid was broken down into women who had never bore a child and were on thyroid over 15 years, those women had a 33 percent excess risk of breast cancer. Women who had children had a 20 percent increased risk of breast cancer by virtue of using thyroid pills over 15 years. The conclusion of this study was that an underactive thyroid treated with thyroid extract for more than 15 years is a breast cancer risk factor.[23]

Diet and Breast Cancer

Following the menopause the incidence of breast cancer in the western culture continues to rise, while in Africa and the Orient the incidence, already low, drops even more to virtually zero in advanced years. The reason for this difference again may be the result

> *An underactive thyroid treated with thyroid extract for more than 15 years is a breast cancer risk factor.*

Fig. 4-4

A High Fat Diet is related to an increased likelihood of breast cancer. Black women have the highest incidence of obesity in this country.

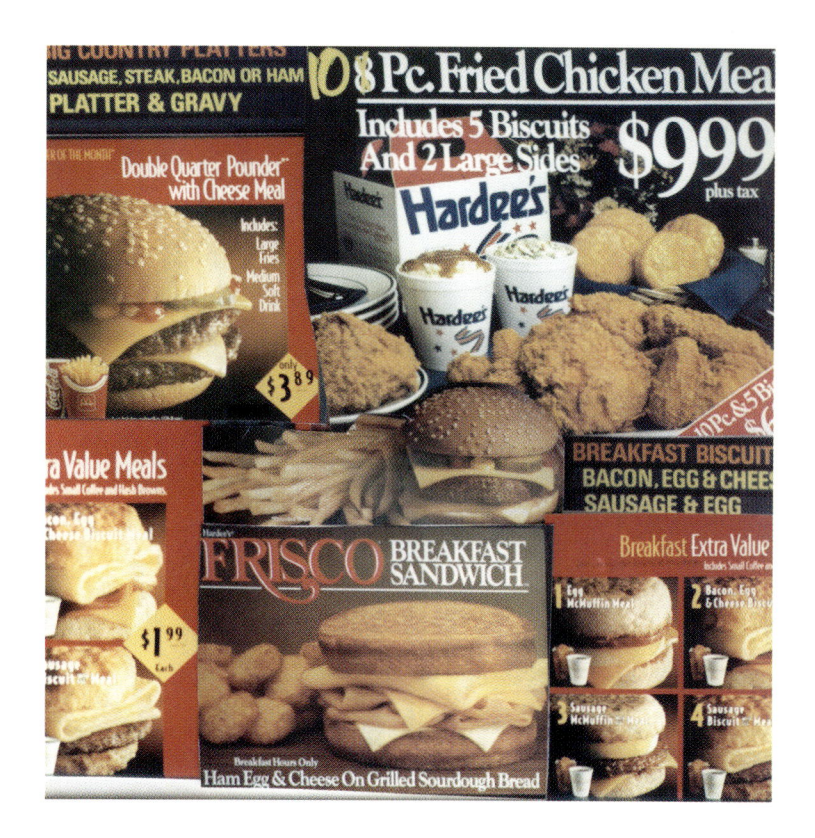

of hormone influence stimulated by the western diet.

It has been shown that fat and obesity are directly related to breast cancer in later years.[24] Other studies correlate body size and breast cancer, and if obesity is associated with hypertension and diabetes the incidence of breast cancer is further increased.[25]

This may help explain why black women are showing an accelerated incidence of breast cancer. Black women are generally larger than white women. In fact American black women have the greatest incidence of obesity in this country—more than black or white males and more than white women.

Earlier I mentioned that **African** black women rarely had breast cancer. It has been demonstrated in South Africa that when the rural black woman moved to the city and assumed the western style high fat diet, the breast cancer rate began to increase sharply over a few years. Another study indicated that if one

Fig. 4-5
Smoking has not been shown to be directly related to breast cancer in most reports. But smoking may aggravate fibrocystic dysplasia.

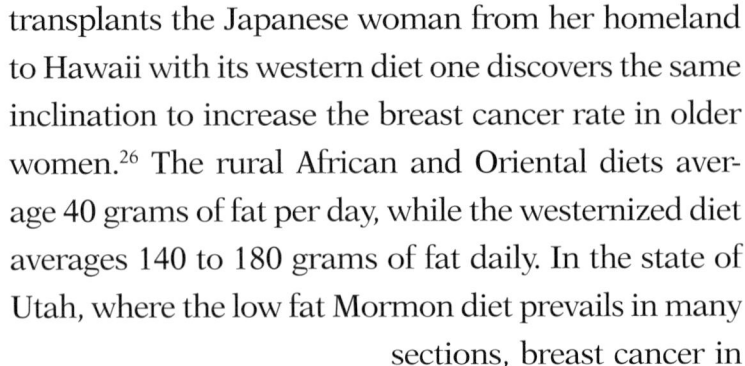

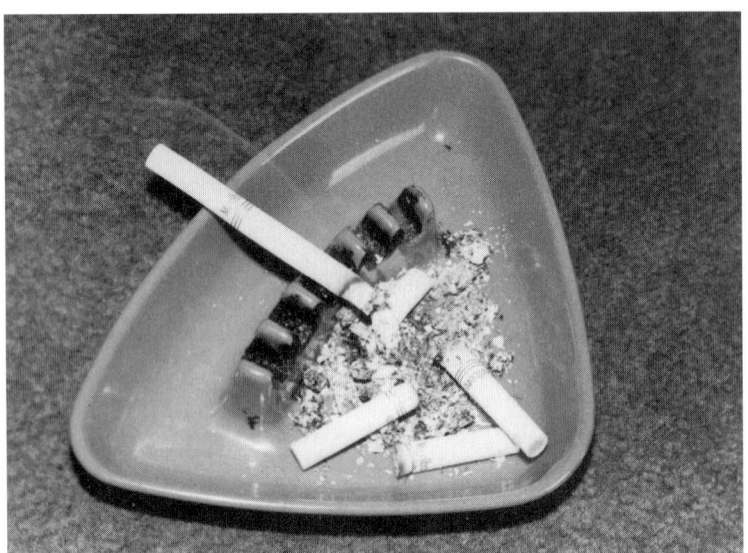

transplants the Japanese woman from her homeland to Hawaii with its western diet one discovers the same inclination to increase the breast cancer rate in older women.[26] The rural African and Oriental diets average 40 grams of fat per day, while the westernized diet averages 140 to 180 grams of fat daily. In the state of Utah, where the low fat Mormon diet prevails in many sections, breast cancer in white women is lower than the national average.[27]

Smoking and Breast Cancer

Most medical studies refute the association of breast cancer and cigarette smoking; although a few reports suggest otherwise. In fact one group examined the question on two occasions. The first study showed that smoking was associated with breast cancer and the second found no correlation whatsoever.[28]

Racial Genetics and Breast Cancer

Among black African women breast cancer is a rarity, but in the United States breast cancer is occurring in epidemic proportions among black women. You might wonder, 'Why this difference? If cancer of the breast is so rare among our black African sisters, why is it so prevalent in American black women? Are we not essentially the same people, or are we so different?'

Well, not only is diet a factor. The fickle finger points emphatically to race. The Negro, if you will, is a hybrid group in the United States that began shortly after the first slaves were brought to America around 1619. The genetic pool of the pure strain black African was blended with the Indian or native American, the Hispanic, and most of all the European white slave master. The Negro hybrid race flourished with continual addition of Caucasian genes during the antebellum era and even unto this day we witness a continued blending of the races.

For a long time we were unable to accurately measure the amount of Caucasian genetic mixture in a population of black Americans. Then someone noted that the whites had more blood type A than blacks.

With this marker one could roughly estimate the degree of Caucasian mixture in a large population of blacks. This was only a very crude supposition since various groups of pure strain Africans had differing amounts of type A blood. Then in 1969 there was a breakthrough of sorts. Dr T. Edward Reed, a Canadian geneticist persuasively demonstrated the usefulness of the Caucasian gene Fa of the Duffy blood group. This so-called Duffy gene is prevalent in all Caucasians and virtually absent in pure strain black Africans.[29]

In fact the gene is exclusively a Caucasian phenomena and if the Duffy gene is found in a population of hybrid Negroes, one could accurately estimate the percentage of Caucasian admixture in that population.

Dr. Reed next examined black people in the northern United States for the presence of the Duffy gene and compared this with the presence of the Duffy gene in a population of southern blacks. He showed that liver cirrhosis due to alcohol abuse was found in whites and only in blacks with the Duffy gene. He predicted that other diseases in Negroes would probably be found in addition to liver cirrhosis that would be tied to the Caucasian admixture.

The following year Dr. Nicholas Petrakis, at the University of California Medical School in San Francisco used Reed's conclusions to examine the incidence of breast cancer in black American women.[30] First he observed that black Ugandans and Nigerians had virtually no trace of the Duffy gene and a breast cancer rate of 9.5 per hundred thousand—an extremely low rate. Then he measured the Duffy gene frequency in American whites and found it to be present in all cases. The breast cancer incidence in white American women in that particular year was 69 per hundred thousand, one of the highest rates in the world. Finally, Dr Petrakis measured the Duffy gene frequency in three populations of black women in Detroit, Atlanta, and Oakland, California. He also measured the frequency of breast cancer in these populations. His findings which were highly significant showed that the northern black women had a greater admixture of the Caucasian Duffy gene and a proportionately greater incidence of breast cancer which corroborated Reed's findings.

In other words he discovered that black populations had more breast cancer, proportional to the extent of the white genetic admixture.

Socio-economic Status and Breast Cancer— Risk or Fate?

Socio-economic status (SES) is a conglomeration of such variables as median family income, years of formal education, percent below the poverty level, and other related measurements. Statisticians have attempted with some success to relate an increased chance for breast cancer with a higher SES. They have gone to some length with statistical machinations to show that women who have a college education, high income, and live in a fancy house have more breast cancer than poor blacks. They have also demonstrated that survival after cancer diagnosis favors those of the higher SES and these are predominantly whites.

I find difficulty with the simplistic notion that education or money actually causes breast cancer; or that simply by the accident of being black condemns one to a poor prognosis. The question is, 'Is survival actually due to SES or is SES simply a marker for some other causative factor.'

On closer scrutiny one finds that the upper crust, who are more often Caucasian, have never born a child or had a first child at an older age. They probably use hormones for one reason or another, and exist on a high fat diet. There's also the predominant estrogen type produced that are carcinogenic. These are all possible risk factors for breast cancer.

As for the poor prognosis for black women, McWhorter and his colleagues reporting in the American Journal of Public Health in 1987 studied 36,905 breast cancer cases.[35] They found that black women with breast cancer received less aggressive treatment. They were most likely to either have no surgery or certainly no cancer-directed treatment. However, this difference was more related to poverty than race. I say it can be related to either since they so often exist together.

A report from the American Cancer Society in 1986 concluded that socio-economic status (SES) rather than race determined survival after cancer diagnosis.[31] If that's the case, then blacks and whites who contract breast cancer and share a similar high socio-

Black populations had more breast cancer, proportional to the extent of the white genetic admixture.

If you are black your prognosis will not be nearly as favorable as your white counterpart.

economic status should likewise share a similar favorable prognosis. **They do not!** If you are black, rich, and educated, your prognosis will not be nearly as favorable as your white counterpart.[32,33]

On the other hand, when looking at other cancers in which blacks have a bad prognosis such as bladder, prostate, and uterus, **race**, undeniably, remains the predominant factor. In a study by Mayer in 1989, it was shown that black patients regardless of SES were more likely to go untreated following a diagnosis of bladder and other cancers with a predictably grave outcome.[36]

An earlier paper by Wynder and his associates in studying only white women showed there was no difference in breast cancer incidence or survival based on SES. In other words poor whites and rich whites contracted breast cancer at the same rate and fared equally after treatment.[34]

An article in the Journal of the National Cancer Institute in 1992 revealed that black women, without considering SES, were more likely to have advanced breast cancer when first diagnosed, with a corresponding high mortality.[37]

Investigators seem to agree that if there is a socioeconomic basis for the dismal outlook for black women, it is the poverty component, borne of racism that appears to be the key.

We know that the entry into the medical marketplace for poor black families is more cumbersome and discouraging. Transportation may be a problem. Fee for service is often out of the question. Even the hours spent in overflowing waiting rooms, beset by cold, indifferent clerks and receptionists, can be a harrowing experience as small children and chores go unattended.

Why the economically disadvantaged should be doomed to a higher mortality has never been answered or squarely confronted. Even when you match the disadvantaged, at whatever stage of disease you find them, against the socio-economically advantaged at a comparable stage of disease, the poor still exhibit a higher mortality.

Why are we losing so many women—poor and black or rich and black for that matter—to breast cancer? I suspect, and the data suggests, that the overall medical care and attention offered this group is less than the optimum—to say the least.

In a society where black infant mortality is almost twice that of white babies and statistics all along the line bear out the racial dichotomy, I would venture that pervasive racism seeping through the medical establishment, frustrates even fundamental efforts of health care delivery to black people.

In 1984 a prestigious Cancer Center in New York informed me (personal correspondence) that they conducted a so-called breast cancer screening program in Harlem using trained palpators to uncover breast lumps. A trained palpator, for your information, is a lay person from the community with no particular medical background, trained for several weeks perhaps, to feel breasts and then introduced to the black community as palpators to uncover cancer.

At the same time these investigators from the Ivory Tower knew that in the hands of the most experienced physicians, half the tumors would be missed by palpation alone. They also knew that mammography in conjunction with careful physical examination is the current recommendation for screening. This was outrageous mis-commitment. Can you imagine a

Black women, without considering SES, were more likely to have advanced breast cancer when first diagnosed, with a corresponding high mortality.

ghetto palpator turned loose on a paying customer in the sacrosanct Ivory Tower? I assume this is not being done in 1993.

Yet in 1993, by and large, it's the crowded inner-city clinics catering to the poor and the black where one finds the most complications and the highest mortality figures in breast cancer and other diseases. In the medical arena as everywhere else in our society, the cannon fodder remains the same. In the foreseeable future, I suspect, the fickle finger will continue to point to the combination 'black and poor' as a **special** risk category in the breast cancer dilemma.

Nevertheless, as we shall read in the next chapter, black women have consistently failed to take advantage of the cancer screening clinics that **are** available for a variety of reasons; and this will require a special ongoing educational effort on the part of all of us.

REFERENCES

1. National Cancer Institute SEER Program 1973-1985

2. NCI Seer Program 1973-1981

3. Young JL Devesa SS Cutler SJ :Incidence of Cancer in united states blacks. Cancer Research 35:Nov 1975 3523-3536

4. MacMahon, Cole P, Brown J: Etiology of human breast cancer: a review. J Natl Cancer Inst 50:21-42 1973

5. Anderson DE :Genetic study of breast cancer: identification of a high risk group. Cancer 34:1090-1097, 1974

6. Robbins G Berg JW :Bilateral primary breast cancer; a prospective clinical pathological study. Cancer 17:1501-1527, 1964

7. MacMahon B, Cole P, Lin TM et al: Age at first birth and breast cancer risk. Bull WHO 43:2909-221, 1970

8. Kamoi M: Statistical study on relation between breast cancer and lactation period. I. A comparative study through cumulative frequency distribution. Tohoku J Exp Med 72: 59-65 1960

9. Brody H, Cullem, M: Carcinoma of breast seventeen years after mammography with thorotrast. Surgery 42:600-606 1957

10. MacKenzie, I: Breast cancer following multiple fluroscopies. Brit J Cancer 19: 1-8, 165

11. Wanebo CK, Johnson, KG, Sato K, Thorslund TW: Breast cancer after exposure to the atomic bombing of hiroshima and nagasaki. NEJM 279:13 Sept 26, 1968 667-671

12. Warren S: The relation of "chronic mastitis" to carcinoma of the breast. SG&O 71:257-278, 1940

13. Black MM Barclay TH Cutler SJ et al: Association of atypical characteristic of benign breast lesions with subsequent risk of breast cancer. Cancer 29:338-343, 1972

14. Lemon HM :Abnormal estrogen metabolism and tissue estrogen receptor proteins in breast cancer. Cancer 25:423-435, 1970

15. Macdonald EJ :Ethnic and Regional Considerations in Epidemiology of breast cancer. J Amer Med Women's Asso 30:3 March 1975

16. Mirra AP Cole P MacMahon B :Breast cancer in an area of high parity; Sao Paulo Brazil. Cancer res.31:77, 1971

17. Lemon HM :Pathophysiologic considerations in the treatment of menopausal patients with estrogens; the role of estriol in the prevention of mammary carcinoma. Acta Endocrinologica 1980 Suppl.233: 17-27

18. Lipsett MB :Hormones, nutrition, and cancer. Cancer Research 35:3359-3361 Nov 1975

19. Henderson BE Gerkins V Rosario I et al :Elevated serum levels of estrogen and prolactin in daughters of patients with breast cancer. NEJM 293:16 790-794 Oct 16 1975

20. Hoover R Gray LA Cole P et al :Menopausal estrogens and breast cancer NEJM 295:8 401-405 Aug 19 1976

21. FasalE Paffenbarger RS :Oral Contraceptives as related to cancer and benign lesions of the breast. J Nat. Cancer Inst 55:4 767-773 Oct 1975

22. Child M Vellios F Meigs JW et al MMWR 31:29 393-394 July 30, 1982

23. Kapdi CC Wolfe JN :Breast cancer relationship to thyroid supplements for hypothyroidism JAMA 236:10 1124-1127 Sept 6, 1976

24. Lipsett MB :Hormones, nutrition, and cancer. Cancer Research 35: 3359-3361

25. deWaard F :Breast cancer incidence and nutritional status with particular reference to body weight and height. Cancer Research 35:3351-3356 Nov1975

26. Dickinson LE MacMahon B Cole P et al :Estrogen Profiles of oriental and caucasian women in hawaii NEJM 291:23 1211-1214 Dec 5, 1974

27. Carroll KK :Experimental evidence of dietary factors and hormone-dependent cancers. Cancer Research35:3374-3383 Nov 1975

28. Schechter MT Miller AB Howe GR et al :Cigarette smoking and breast cancer: case control studies of prevalent and incident cancer in the Canadian National Breast Screening Study. Am J Epidemiol 1989 Aug;130(2):213-220

29. Reed TE :Caucasian genes in american negroes. Science 165:762-768 Aug 22, 1969

30. Petrakis NL :Some preliminary observations on the influence of genetic admixture on cancer incidence in american negroes. Int J Cancer 7:256-258 1971

31. American Cancer Society:Special Report on Cancer in the Economically disadvantaged, prepared by the Amer Can

Soc, Sub comm on Can in the Economically Disadvantaged. New York, Amer Can Society, 1986

32. Bain RP Greenberg RS Whitaker JP :Racial differences in survival of women with breast cancer. J Chronic Dis 39:631-642, 1986

33. Ragland KE Selvin S Merrill DW : Black-white differences in stage specific cancer survival: Analysis of seven selected sites. Am J Epdemiol 133:672-682, 1991

34. Wynder EL MacCornack FA Stellman SD :The epidemology of breast cancer in 785 united states caucasian women. Cancer 41:6 June 1978 2341-2353

35. McWhorter WP Mayer WJ :Blac/white differences in type of initial breast cancer treatment and implications for survival. Am J Public Health 1987 Dec ;77 (12):1515-7

36. Mayer WJ McWhorter WP Black/white differences in non-treatment of bladder cancer patients and implications for survival. Am J Public Health 1989 Jun;79(6):772-5

37. Coates RJ Bransfield DD Wesley M et al :Differences between black and white women with breast cancer in time from symptom recognition to medical consultation. Black/White survival study group. J Natl Cancer Inst (1992 Jun 17) 84(12):938-50

38. Garfinkel L: Current Trends in Breast Cancer. CA-A Can. J Phys.43:1 Jan/Feb 1993 pp 5-6.

39. Olsson H Moller TR Ranstam J: Early oral contraceptive use and breast cancer among premomenopausal women: Final report from a study in southern Sweden. J Natl Cancer 1989;8

40. McDivitt RW Stevens JA Lee NC et al: Cancer and steroid hormone study group....Cancer 1992; 69:1408-14

41. White E: Rising incidence of breast cancer (response to letter).JNCI 80:2, 1988

42. Muss HB Hunter CP Wesley M et al: Treatment Plans for Black and White Women......: Cancer 70:2460-2467, 1992

"Education, income, and health insurance status are more important in determining the likelihood of receiving screening mammography than race" (according to Dr Victor G Vogel, MD, MHS, Assistant Professor of Medicine and Epidemiology-Department of Medical Oncology-The University of Texas, MD Anderson Cancer Center in Houston, Texas). This is an example of doublespeak. Tell me, who is most educationally deprived, who is disproportionately poor, and who is most likely to be without health insurance. Black folks! And guess who is less likely to have a mammogram. You!

CHAPTER FIVE

A NEEDLE IN THE HAYSTACK
Finding Breast Cancer

*d*iscovering breast cancer in the general population is like finding a needle in a haystack. For the private sector it would be impractical, if not impossible, to screen the entire country on a regular basis. This is clearly a matter for government to address, like any other public health issue, since it must be continuous and ongoing. Presently there is little government funding available. Certainly there is only mediocre commitment.

Nevertheless, early attempts by the private sector to screen women for breast cancer on a large scale have been recorded. It began in the 1950's when x-ray mammography was not part of the screening process, only breast palpation and observation were done.[1] Investigators showed that breast cancer could be discovered in an early stage. Whether or not this increased the cure rate or just prolonged survival could not be said with certainty since there was no control group for comparison. To justify the time and public expense of large scale screening, it was imperative to prove that breast cancer mortality could be significantly reduced by comparing the results to a control group.

Blacks underestimate the prevalence of cancer and are less aware of cancer's warning signs.

• • • • • • •

The first time such a control group was used for comparison was done by the Breast Cancer Screening Project of the Health Insurance Plan of Greater New York. This study commonly called the HIP project was begun in December 1963.[2] A population of women numbering 62,000, aged 40 to 64 was gleaned from the insurance registry and divided into two equal groups. These groups were closely matched with regards to age, marital status, number of children, benign breast disease, religion, and even education. No mention of race was made.

One group was screened for breast cancer in a periodic systematic manner, and the control group received only their customary medical attention. The screened group was examined yearly for cancer that could be discovered by x-ray mammography or physical examination. Women were also instructed in breast self examination. In 1972 after nine years of screening the HIP project reported a 30 percent less mortality from breast cancer in the screened group, when compared to the control group. Of the cancers found in the screened group, 33 percent were discovered only by mammography and 45 percent found by palpation alone. If the population was divided according to age groups, only 19 percent of cases in the 40-49 age category could be found by mammography alone. In the 50-59 age group, mammography alone was successful in 42 percent of cases. This finding was explained on the basis of the greater density of breast tissue in the younger women and the shortcomings of the x-ray equipment used in the 1960's. In the following decades using selinium plates and better equipment the mammogram yield would dramatically improve.

After the HIP project findings, the medical profession began to seriously speculate that finding the needle in the hay stack was feasible, and clinicians around the country geared up for a massive screening to find hidden breast cancer. Nevertheless there were many hindrances. For one thing getting asymptomatic women, particularly black women, to come in for an examination and return periodically required much effort in solicitation and follow-up. There was no existing list of women from which to draw as in the HIP study. Another problem was cost effectiveness. The sheer number of medical personnel and support services to conduct the exams, compile the data, and analyze the statistics could prove to be a formidable task.

Would it be economically feasible to find the needle in the haystack working through the private sector?

A screening project was set up by the Guttman Institute in New York in 1968, headed by Dr. Philip Strax.[3] Dr Strax, designed his project to answer questions concerning feasibility of operation and cost effectiveness. The project was prepared to screen 50,000 women per year with an additional 15,000 screened through mobile units and out-reach programs. Not only were they supported by charitable gifts; but the American Cancer Society, New York Division, and the National Cancer Institute lent their combined assistance.

Using a new generation of mammographic machines and films, Dr Strax and his associates were impressed with the capacity of mammography and physical examination to uncover cancers independently. When using these two modalities together, 95 percent of cancers were found on the initial screening. They also noted that women re-screened after only a year interval would show a cancer not previously picked up. It was estimated that 5 to 10 percent of unsuspected breast cancers were missed even with excellent screening technique. Those missed should be discovered within a year by re-examination or by the patient herself discovering the suspicious lesions in the interim.

Dr Strax found that the needs of an adequate screening project could be enormous. Some of the financial burden, however, could be curtailed by replacing doctors, and nurses with health aides. These aides, some taken from the community served, were trained to carry out the entire project under proper supervision. The new mammography machines were simple in their design and required only a few weeks to master. A technician, it was learned, could be fully trained in about 4 weeks to begin breast inspection and palpation. It was shown that a technician, working with hundreds of mammograms learned to spot the abnormal films quite handily. Out of a hundred films they would call ten abnormal. Almost always if a cancer was present in the hundred films, it would be in the ten chosen for further scrutiny. A cadre of vocational nurses and nurses aides were ideal for this purpose. This saved the trained physician-radiologist valuable time, and it was obviously cost-effective for the project. After five years, the cost was calculated to be approximately twenty dollars per patient.

Dr Strax and others began to realize that if the purpose of mass screening is to lower the death rate of breast cancer patients, then this must clearly be a public health issue that should be supported by public health tax dollars. Ah, But there's the rub.

Fifty one percent of black women in 1980 believed that exposing breast cancer to air during surgery would cause spread of the malignancy.
● ● ● ● ● ● ●

As you can imagine the public trough is crowded with many other worthy health causes—each vying for a preferential pecking order. Multiple sclerosis, The Heart Fund, Hypertension Screening, Maternal and Child Welfare, Drug Abuse, and now the AIDS epidemic—all depend in large measure on public funding.

Whenever a new program is evaluated for financial assistance the cost/benefit ratio is paramount. The cost effectiveness is uppermost in the mind of the bureaucrat holding the purse strings; and at this point too little government monies have been expended to support voluntary groups in breast cancer screening, such as the Guttman Institute project.

The Guttman project was supported by the American Cancer Society volunteers who used the media (radio and print) to advertise that breast screening was available. Only 5.3 percent of those responding to the call for free breast screening were black women, numbering 14,864. Of that number 43.1 percent completed the five year screening, compared to 53 percent of the white women. In fact, after the first two annual exams, 32.6 percent of the black women had dropped out of the program, compared to 23.9 percent of the white group.

Even with this poor attendance breast cancer was found in 5.9 percent of the black women and 5.4 percent of the whites. Similar cancer detection rates between the races continued over the five year period in spite of the fact that so many black women didn't bother to come back each year. We can only speculate on how many black women with breast cancer were missed because they did not return for follow-up. As it turned out, 80 percent of the breast cancers that were detected during the five year period were very early and probably curable. This is twice the percent of black women who turn up at clinics and medical offices with early breast cancer.[4]

The largest screening program for breast cancer to date was reported in 1988. Two hundred eighty thousand women were screened over a five year period under the auspices of The National Cancer Institute and The American Cancer Society. They joined forces and organized the Breast Cancer Detection Demonstration Project (BCDDP).[5]

They initially funded 29 centers throughout the country that began to screen women for breast cancer. The program was designed to screen a population of women annually for five years and then to follow them for an additional five years. Statistics from this effort showed that 41.6 percent of the cancers uncovered were found by mammography alone while physical examination alone found 8.7 percent. One third of cancers found were fifty years of age or younger. Unfortunately women under age forty were excluded.

In the HIP project of the 1960's, mammography alone detected about 30 percent of the cancers and fifty percent were detected by physical ex-

DETECTING BREAST CANCER

1. Women 20 years of age and older should perform breast self-examination every month.
2. Women 20 to 40 years of age should have physical examination of the breast every three years, and women over 40 should have a physical examination of the breast every year.
3. Women at age 40 should have a baseline mammogram *(the baseline was originally 35 years of age).*
4. Women between the ages of 40 and 50 should have a mammogram every two years.
5. Women over age 50 should have a mammogram every year when feasible.
6. Women must consult their personal physician or clinic regarding the frequency of mammography in cases where there is a strong family history.

amination alone.[6] This difference is a result of the strides made in mammography which is now considered the major tool in finding very early unsuspected breast cancers.

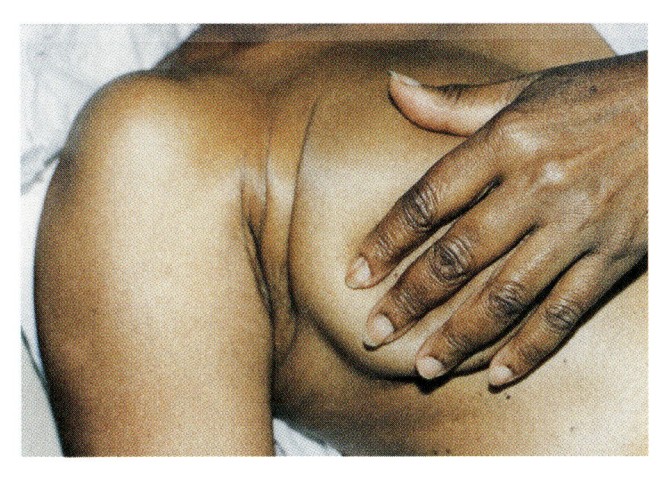

Fig. 5-1
Breast Self Examination (BSE) should be taught by your health provider or public health facility. Self breast examination on a monthly basis must start at age 20.

The BCDDP was a noble endeavor. However, it only scratched the surface. With the resources now at our disposal it is simply not feasible for private clinics to screen such a huge target population on a regular basis. The hay stack is too great, the needle too small, and the searchers too few.

Consequently, all women, black and white must seek relief in the political arena. With the available technology now at our disposal, 30 percent more women could be saved; the needle could be found if we were politically committed.

As a direct result of the BCDDP, the American Cancer Society in 1988 joined with 12 national organizations including the predominantly black National Medical Association to issue specific guidelines for detecting breast cancer in asymptomatic women. The most pertinent suggestions are presented on page 92.

In certain cases of a strong family history of breast cancer, that is, cancer occurring before age 30, The first degree relatives such as mother, daughters and sisters, have a 50% chance of early onset of breast cancer. For these women it is suggested that BSE begin at age fifteen and biennial mammography begin at age twenty, and then yearly at age thirty-five.[12]

By the same token **young** black women have

proven to be at special risk.[13] **For all black women, I suggest, in addition to early BSE, that a baseline mammogram be done between the age of 30 and 35, and then yearly thereafter.** Because of the density of the breast in these young women, mammography is 20 to 25 percent less effective. Though there is no doubt that cancers will be found, there will not be nearly as many cases as in older age groups. So the cost of each cancer found will be high. But think of the total number of productive years that can be added to the lives of those young women.

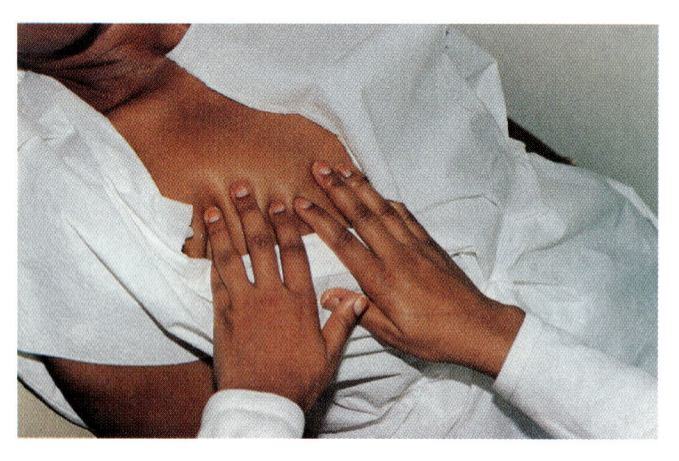

If every woman age 20 and over would take it upon herself to follow these guidelines and urge friends and loved ones to also seek out screening programs, breast cancer would be discovered at a curable stage, often before a lump was palpable.

Many clinics following the Guttman Institute lead have opened their doors to earnestly seek out early breast cancer—for a price. But they are only seeing the tip of the iceberg, and many do not serve the needs of black and poor women because of their location, budgetary guidelines, etc. Another important factor to remember is that many black women don't even know these clinics exist.

Consequently, we must aggressively direct a keen dedicated offensive towards that population that appears to encompass the majority of women who succumb to breast cancer: the least informed. This would mean a special effort in the black commu-

Fig. 5-2
Anything Suspicious should be verified by your health provider. insist on a mammogram. If you have any doubt, get another medical opinion.

nity where no information and mis-information reign supreme.

Figures released by the National Cancer Institute indicate that during the five year period 1973 through 1977, the incidence of breast cancer increased 28 percent among black women compared to 18 percent among whites.[7] This trend of increased frequency of breast cancer among black women is continuing.

Surveys conducted by the American Cancer Society in 1980 indicated that American black women are less exposed to cancer information than white women.[8] Lower income black women are less likely to perform breast self-examination. Blacks underestimate the prevalence of cancer and are less aware of cancer's warning signs. Although black and white women think of breast cancer when speaking generally of cancer only 30 percent of blacks had heard of a mammogram (x-ray) examination of the breast, compared to 53 percent of white women. Fifty one percent of black women in the 1980 survey believed that exposing the cancer to air during surgery would cause spread of the malignancy. None of the white women questioned believed this myth.

The survey also showed that twice as many black women as white women voiced their desire not to be told they had cancer if it were true; and 59 percent of blacks believed that getting cancer is an automatic death sentence compared to only 36 percent of whites. Hopefully these misconceptions have changed in the ensuing decade.

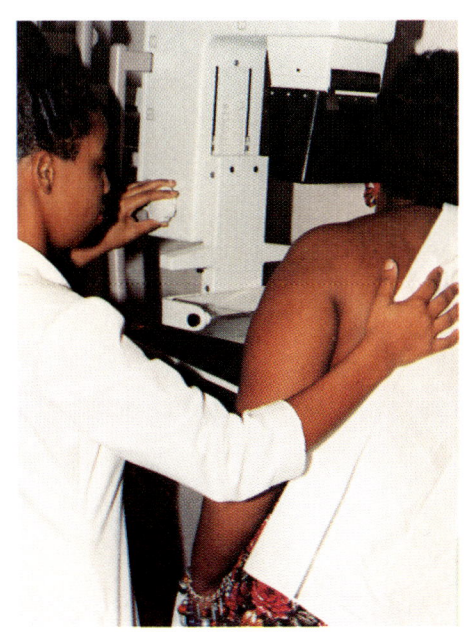

In 1988 health care screening specialists came together to discuss ways and means of getting more

Fig. 5-3
Sreening Mammography should be a part of every local health department. Technicians can be trained in four weeks to perform mammography.

women screened for breast cancer. Like most of these 'study groups' there was no real action because there was no real commitment for funding.[9] Here we have one of the most readily diagnosed and treatable cancers in the spectrum being studied ad infinitum, The issue that can make a difference—funding—is given lip service—talked to death and then put on the shelf until the next talk-a-thon.

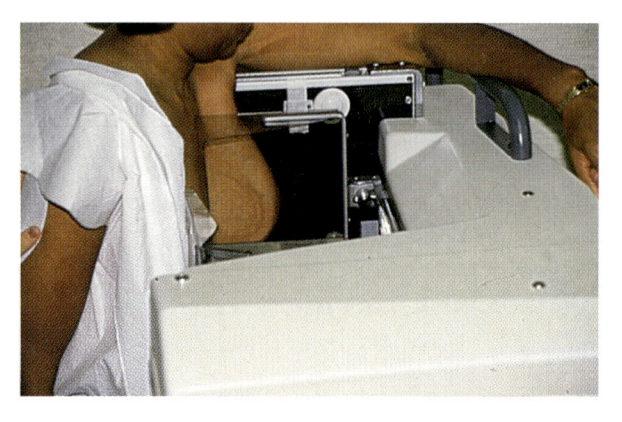

Breast cancer screening should be an integral part of every health department in every community. If they can provide free immunization for measles and mumps, they can provide mammography free of charge. It's simply a matter of demand and creating commitment. The reason we don't have those screening facilities along with an overall adequate health care systems is because the politician is not responsive.

Politics is the ability to shape public policy and consensus through the legislative process. It's about wielding power to get things done. It's an art form—a craft, a special talent. I don't have that talent; but I wouldn't be surprised if there's someone reading this chapter right now who **does** have that kind of organizational skill to pull it off. I'm sure, some of you readers know how to get things done. Politics is the art of squeaking the wheel and getting the oil. Some of you even have access to the ear of friends in high places.

If an articulate (or not so articulate) group of black women showed up at the local health department fired up and committed, on a regular basis there would be some action. In fact I bet if only a

Fig. 5-4
Mammography Technicians can also be trained to screen for cancer or suspicious lesions which should be verified by a radiologist. This has been done in massive screening programs with good results.

If an articulate (or not so articulate) group of black women showed up at the local health department fired up and committed, on a regular basis there would be some action.

• • • • • • •

few **choice** sisters marched there'd be a positive response. The answer is pure and simple. If you want to find the needle in the haystack, then it's up to you to start digging.

Gear up for a massive ongoing effort of education and awareness in your community in order to somehow come to grips with this epidemic. Screening and education working in harmony form a winning combination for maximum results.

There have been local efforts on the state level such as that done in Wisconsin which showed that detection of breast cancer increased simply by instigating a breast cancer awareness program.[10] Similar efforts in other parts of the country have also had some success.[11] Recently the Breast Cancer Coalition has had some success in bringing the need for funding to the attention of President Clinton.

Until Public Health catches up, private screening clinics must open their doors to the uninsured and the have-nots. In Montgomery, Alabama, some hospitals and private breast screening clinics open their doors to the uninsured once a year for little or no cost to the patient. This proves that this epidemic can be fought and controlled by medical people of goodwill. I consider participation in this endeavor every October an opportunity to be part of something redemptive. If an early cancer is found, then the practice and art of medicine is somehow justified—it becomes a noble business again. Being a physician must be more than just making a good living. Like Arthur Ashe said: 'Getting makes a living, ...giving makes a life'.

Black leaders in the medical profession must join others in getting across a message that is crystal clear. The public and the politicians must understand: Breast cancer can be detected early in a practical, cost efficient way. Through monthly breast self-examination, periodic medical examination, and mammography screening—incredulous though it may seem, the needle in the hay stack can be found!

REFERENCES

1. Holleb AI, Venet L, Day E: Breast cancer detected by routine physical examination. NY State H Med 60:823-827 1960

2. Shapiro S Strax P Venet L :Periodic breast cancer screening. Arch Environ. Health 15:547-553, 1967

3. Strax P The Guttman Institute story. In: Strax P ed Control of Breast Cancer Through Mass Screening. Littleton, Massachusetts PSG Publishing Co., 1979; 183-187

4. Shapiro S, Venet L, Strax P: Prospects for eliminating racial difference in breast cancer survival rates. A J Pub H 72:10 1142-1145 Oct 1982

5. Breslow L: Final reports of national cancer institute ad hoc working group on mammography screening for breast cancer and a summary report of their joint findings and recommendations. Epidemiology-biostatistics working group. DHEW Publication No. (NIH) 77-1400 Washington D C: Govt Print Office, 1977

6. Strax P, Venet L, Shapiro S: Mass screening in mammary cancer. 23:875-878 April 1969

7. National Cancer Institute SEER Program 1973-1981

8. Black americans' attitudes toward cancer and cancer tests: Highlights of a study. Ca-Cancer J for Clinicians 31:4 July/Aug 1981

9. Dodd GR Fink DJ Murphy GP :Breast cancer detection and community practice: Executive summary report of a workshop cosponsored by the general motors cancer research foundation and the american cancer society. Ca-Cancer J for Clinicians 39:4 July/Aug 1989

10. Remington PL Lantz PM :Using apopulation-based cancer reporting system to evaluate a breast cancer detection and awareness program. Ca-Cancer J for Clinicians 42:6 November/December 1992

11. Kaufmam AJ Worrell J Bain RS et al: American cancer society's breast cancer detection awareness program: the 1988 middle tennessee experience. Sout Med J 83:618-620,1990

12. Lynch HT, Fitzgibbons, Lynch, JF: Heterogeneity and Natural History of Hereditary Breast Cancer. Surg Clin of No Amer 70:4 Aug 1990 753-776 13. White E: Rising incidence of breast cancer (response to letter).JNCI 80:2, 1988

CHAPTER SIX

NO NEWS IS GOOD NEWS–RIGHT? WRONG!
Know your Enemy to Survive

You and I fear cancer because it brings suffering and death. In fact we tend to deny any sickness as long as possible. We run from illness like the Boston marathon. It's just human nature to avoid realities that might be unpleasant. As for a check up. Forget it. We don't want any blood tests or even a chest x-ray. Who wants bad news? No news is good news. Right? And so we wait for pain or some disability to goad us to the doctor; and then we hope for some miracle or some good report to speed us on our way, to await the next signal of pain.

Most physicians like me are just like you. We're all in the same bag. Some doctors drink too much, eat too much, and some of us are still smoking. We doctors fail to get check ups, too.

Well, let me be a Baptist preacher for a moment and tell you what I think is right, not what I necessarily do. If you're walking around **knowing** you have a lump in your breast, you should seek medical help. However, if you're putting it off, because of fear, you're not the only one. You've got lots of company. Seventy-five percent of American women rank breast cancer as their number one health fear as noted by The Opinion Research Corporation of Princeton, New Jersey. Fear is a natural reaction to breast cancer or any lump in the breast. And it's hard to go in for a mammogram. It's easy to put it off. How many men over 40 actually get a rectal exam to check for prostate trouble every year? They probably reason just like you and me: 'It doesn't hurt so what's the hurry? Anyway, who want's bad new? No new is good news. Right?' Perhaps not. Ignorance may be bliss, but when it comes to breast cancer you may miss an opportunity for cure, simply by not acting responsibly. Sometimes bad news can turn out okay if it's dealt with in a timely manner. So do your best to take control and direct old man fear to trigger you towards some positive action.

A positive response would be to learn as much as you can about breast cancer now. Know your enemy! Learn how breast cancer can be controlled, and even cured in its early stages. Check with the Public Health Department in your community. Call your doctor or clinic and inquire about available information. A number of pamphlets can be obtained through the Department of Health and Human Services; and the American Medical Association will provide cancer information at a nominal cost. No news is not good news. It's ignorance.

Another good source of information, mostly free for the asking, is provided through the local chapter of the American Cancer Society.

Films and speakers are available for groups to stimulate discussion and answer questions. There is too much misinformation circulating in our community. These agencies will welcome your questions and input in designing a presentation for your church group or club.

Ignorance may be bliss, but when it comes to breast cancer you may miss an opportunity for cure, simply by not acting responsibly.

> **M**ost physicians agree that breast cancer is a disease in which the patient is expected to participate in learning about the types of breast cancer and the implications for care.
> • • • • • • •

For diagnosis and treatment it may be advisable to seek out a comprehensive cancer clinic if you live in a metropolitan center. These clinics are part of every university medical center, and free-standing breast centers are springing up in cities and towns across the nation. Be sure the facility has state of the art equipment and a certified radiologist to interpret the x-rays.

The Office of Cancer Communications, National Cancer Institute, Bethesda, MD, would be able to direct you to a center near your home. Other sources to explore include The National Black Women's Health Project, The Breast Cancer Resources Committee, or the Breast Cancer Coalition.

Every woman should develop the capacity to suspect the breast cancer intruder in the very early months before invasion. With some familiarity with the different stages of breast cancer and even the microscopic patterns as they pertain to prognosis, a patient can help herself towards wellness by appreciating the facts of her case; and thus be more inclined to cooperate with the treatment program outlined by her doctor. Most physicians agree that breast cancer is a disease in which the patient is expected to participate in learning about the types of breast cancer and the implications for care.

The following discussion is included to help answer some questions for readers who wish a more in-depth discussion. You may find it too detailed and you may wish to skip over it and go on to Chapter 7—The Battle Plan.

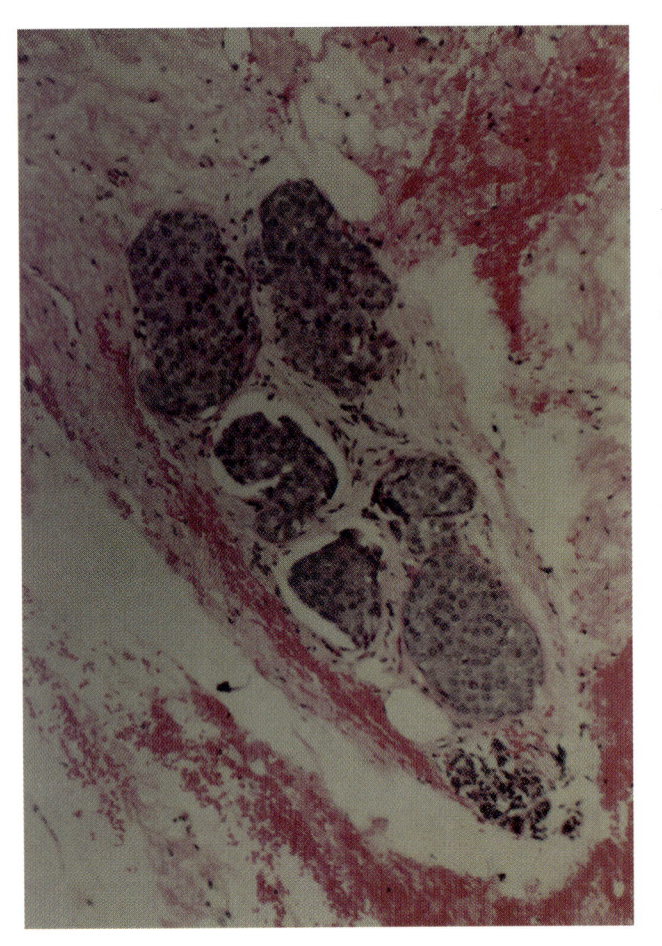

HISTOLOGY (CELLULAR PATTERN)

Every type of breast cancer can be classified by its peculiar pattern of malignant cells as viewed through the microscope. Each type of cancer has it's own distinctive growth idiosyncrasy that bears on treatment options and ultimate survival. Two breast cancers of the same size may have entirely different potentials for local extension and dissemination. In some types the breast cancer is aggressive and spreads early while other cancers tend to develop slowly and have less propensity to metastasize even when the primary tumor is fairly bulky.[1]

FIG. 6-1
DUCTAL CARCINOMA INSITU (DCIS). This biopsy done in 1993 showed DCIS, a tumor that would eventually become invasive cancer. The purple cells are cancer. Removal of the breast was the patient's option. However, lumpec-tomy may be sufficient according to some authorities with removal of axillary nodes and careful follow-up.

Dr Edwin Fisher of the University of Pittsburgh Medical School showed that ultimate prognosis depends not only on the extent of spread of the cancer when first detected, but also on the cellular type involved. **He named six major cellular types that have different survival implications. These include Ductal, (infiltrating and in situ), Lobular (infiltrating and in situ), Medullary, Mucinous, Tubular, and Combination.**[3]

Infiltrating Ductal

Fifty percent of all breast cancers can be recognized as Infiltrating Ductal. In some series as many as 75 percent are classified as Infiltrating Ductal. If we

FIG. 6-2
INFILTRATING DUCTAL CARCINOMA. This is a serious cancer and removal of lymph nodes was manda-tory. One lymph node revealed spread of the cancer. No physical evidence of distal cancer spread was found. This black woman, 48 years old, had never had a screening mammography. She received a course of chemotherapy after masectomy; but there was no arm swelling or hair loss.

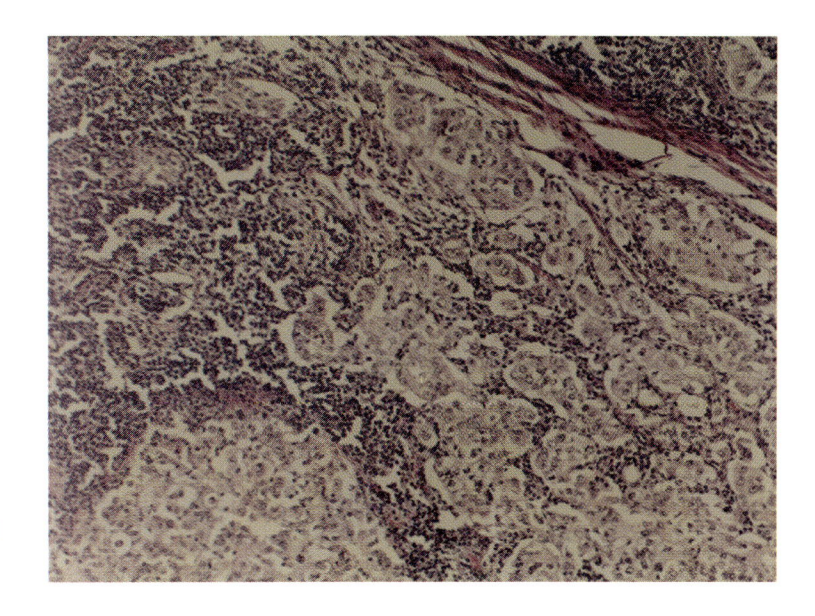

disregard the extent of spread and look at all cases with this cellular pattern, we find that 60 percent will not be cured.

Lobular Infiltrating

The Lobular infiltrative type on the other hand, accounts for only 6 percent of the cancer cell types and the prognosis is better. Thirty percent will be treatment failures.

Lobular Insitu

Then there is the Lobular insitu cancer (LCIS). It is confined to a lobule and has not begun to invade or infiltrate the surrounding normal breast tissue. It occurs in 3 percent of breast cancer cases and is generally found by mammogram before it is palpable. Total mastectomy is usually recommended, because LCIS is a marker indicating that other cancers are very likely to occur in multiple sites (multi-centric) of the breast. The opposite breast (contralateral) may also be involved. Simple mastectomy of the involved breast and close observation of the contralateral breast would seem to be reasonable treatment; but in some cases the opposite breast is also removed.[2]

Medullary, Mucinous, or Tubular

Approximately five percent of all cases of breast cancer will be either the Medullary, Mucinous or Tubular type with a moderate prognosis. The failure rate is 27 percent, discounting the stage. In early cases the prognosis is excellent with less than a 7 percent treatment failure.

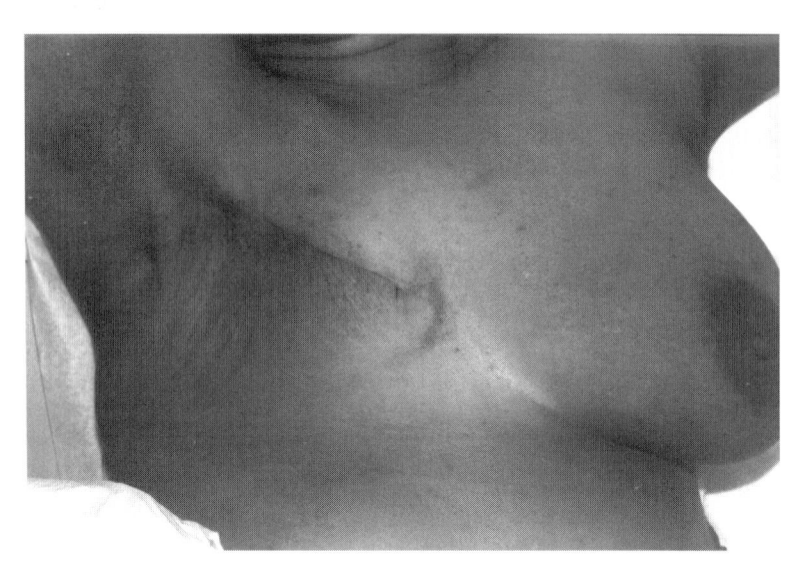

Combination Group

A final histologic cancer type cited by Dr Fisher is the Combination group. In this situation more than one histologic pattern is found in the same cancer. These are mostly Infiltrating Ductal and Tubular, or Infiltrating Ductal and Lobular (invasive) combinations. Occasionally, Mucinous and other rare types are associated with Infiltrating Ductal. The treatment failure rate in the Combination group is 25 percent.

Paget's Disease and Inflammatory Breast Cancer

Two unusual breast cancers, classified under Infiltrating Ductal, should be emphasized since they can be readily detected. They are Paget's Disease, and Inflammatory Cancer.

Paget's Disease is first detected as a rash over the nipple that slowly creeps out over the areola. It looks like an ordinary irritation, After a week or so of home

FIG. 6-3
MODIFIED RADICAL MASTECTOMY WITH AXILLARY DISSECTION. This patient has recovered from surgery and has made an excellent adjustment. Family has been supportive and her husband has remained attentive. Plastic reconstruction was rejected as an option in favor of a prosthesis worn in the bra. Chance for cure is estimated at 60 percent.

> *Paget's Disease is first detected as a rash over the nipple. It looks like an ordinary irritation.*
> •••••••

remedies, a patient may visit her family physician or a dermatologist who may prescribe a cream for the rash that, of course, doesn't work. In disgust the woman may disregard her return appointment to the dermatologist and seek out another physician after several weeks. That doctor may prescribe an antibiotic ointment, wasting precious time. The wiser patient would have either returned to the dermatologist or informed the second physician that creams and ointments had not helped after a few weeks of trial. Undoubtedly, with this history either physician would have suggested a biopsy under local anesthesia. A tiny fragment of skin the size of a pin-head would tell the story. Paget's Disease represents only 2.5 percent of all breast cancers. The typical rash is usually found before a tumor is palpable under the nipple. If treated early about 70 percent will be cured.

Inflammatory breast cancer which is uniformly fatal is extremely rare. It begins as a dusky redness in the dependent part of the breast and simulates mastitis or the inflamed breast of the nursing mother. Although the cancer is incurable life can be extended with early therapy.

Another term you may hear to describe a breast cancer is **comedo carcinoma**, usually associated with the infiltrating ductal type. Comedo means there is an accumulation of cancer cells in the ducts surrounding areas of debris with severe local infiltration of the neighboring tissue.

Not only cellular type but the capacity to infiltrate into surrounding tissue affects prognosis. If veins and lymph channels near the primary cancer are clogged with cancer cells, the recurrent rate is high. Also the size of the lesion is significant. Dr Fisher found that cancers 5 centimeters or larger have metastasized when first discovered, even if the lymph nodes seem to be uninvolved.

Location of the tumor in the breast has implications for the direction of spread. Most cancers occur in the upper outer quadrant with spread into the lymph nodes of the axilla. Tumors that arise in the medial half of the breast also tend to metastasize to the axilla. However, a significant percent will spread medially and infiltrate the internal mammary nodes.

STAGING BREAST CANCER

The most often used method of classifying breast cancer is according to the size of the tumor and the extent of spread to regional lymph nodes and beyond these confines.[4] Also, to be considered, is whether the lesion involves the skin or has penetrated to be fixed to the underlying muscle. With this information one is able to stage the cancer according to the TNM System (Tumor size, Nodes, Metastasis). This TNM System was devised in 1973 by the American Joint Committee for Cancer Staging and End Results. There are four Stages in the TNM System and the prognosis worsens with an increase

STAGING BREAST CANCER

STAGE I T=Breast tumor of any size up to 5 centimeters, minimal skin involvement, no muscle or chest wall attachment. N=No axillary nodes palpable. M=No distant metastasis.

STAGE II T=Same as Stage I. N=One or more nodes palpable in the axilla. M=No distant metastasis.

STAGE III T=Breast tumor over 5 centimeters. N=Same as Stage II plus one or more of the following: Skin ulceration, skin edema, pectoral muscle attachment, nodes fixed in the axilla.

STAGE IV Spread of cancer beyond the axilla (distant metastasis to bone, lung, brain, liver, etc).

> **B**ut this overview will help you to ask specific questions of your doctor. Inquire about the cell type that was found and what that means with regards to your treatment and prognosis.
> • • • • • • •

in the Stage number.

In recent years the TNM System has been criticized for its shortcomings and inaccuracies. At best it is only a very rough guide. The microscopic delineation and estrogen receptor status and other more sophisticated tests are much better prognostic indicators.

Nevertheless, treatment options to a great extent are based upon the following Stage classification.

Some clinicians consider a cancer over 2 centimeters in greatest diameter a Stage II even if there are no axillary nodes positive; and if the cancer is over 5 centimeters, regardless of the axillary node status, the patient is considered a Stage III.

Regardless of admitted imperfection, Staging serves as a useful guide in designing treatment protocols and answering questions concerning prognosis. For example, a patient with Stage I with treatment has an 80 percent chance of surviving ten years or more. A woman in Stage II can expect a 60 percent survival rate at ten years, while a Stage III cancer patient would expect only a 30 percent chance of living free of disease for ten years. These figures can improve depending on the cellular type of cancer involved. Also life can be extended for months and years through various treatment modalities.

I can't expect you to remember all the cellular types of breast cancer. The pathologist (physician who looks at the tissue under the microscope) knows the cellular classifications, and most surgeons also have some familiarity with the various types. Many surgeons insist on seeing the microscopic sections and having the pathologists point out the highlights of the cancer that allow the classification.

But this overview will help you to ask specific questions of your doctor. If a breast biopsy shows the cancer enemy lurking along a duct or infiltrating the normal tissue, inquire about the cell type that was found and what that means with regards to your treatment and prognosis. What was the size of the tumor? Over 5 centimeters? Under 2 centimeters? What section of the breast was the cancer located and were any lymph nodes positive for cancer?

There is data suggesting that the location of the cancer in the breast, whether it be near the breast bone or the armpit, has little or no bearing on the prognosis or curability. Nevertheless, some investigators believe that cancers near the midline require radiation. Ask your doctor his understanding of this controversy.

Then there is the question of blood type and prognosis. British doctors reported in 1970 that women with breast cancer with a blood type of B or AB had a significantly higher incidence and recurrence rate than women with blood type A or O. More recently investigators have not found such a relationship.[5,6]

You may also wish to know if the cancer is estrogen-receptor positive and/or progesterone-receptor positive? These receptor tests on the cancerous tissue that is removed will be discussed further in Chapter Seven. Also be sure a DNA Histogram is done on any biopsy tissue. You don't have to know the definition of aneuploidy or the meaning oncogenes, but ask your doctor to help you know your prognosis—to give you some idea of the aggressiveness of the cancer.[7]

Even if you can't remember the details of the tests and tumor types, ask anyway. 'What kind of tumor do I have? What were the results of the DNA histogram and the ER and PR tests? How does this affect my prognosis and the treatment program? What are my options regarding chemotherapy? And what about

Ask 'what kind of tumor do I have? What were the results of the DNA histogram and the ER and PR tests? How does this affect my prognosis and the treatment program?'

> *You've got to know the cancer enemy to enhance your opportunity for survival; and you must participate in decisions of treatment.*
> ● ● ● ● ● ● ●

Tamoxifen?' Your surgeon will know you're concerned and will answer all questions to your satisfaction. In fact he'll work a little harder in your behalf. You've got to know the cancer enemy to enhance your opportunity for survival; and you must participate in decisions of treatment.

On the other hand many women have little desire to know the details of the disease or the outline of any proposed treatment regimen. Maybe the only news that interests you is simply some indication of your chances of cure. You may want to leave the details to your doctor and his discussions with your family. You may need time to sort things out, to regroup so to speak. Most women, in my experience, eventually come to terms with the disease; and, at some point, expect and appreciate an explanation of treatment alternatives based on the Stage of disease and the histologic type. But everyone at her own pace and her own needs.

Becoming familiar with all aspects of the breast cancer will not only help you to understand the danger, but will stress the need for an early counterattack.

In the next chapter I'll turn to the counterattack and discuss the weapons we have on hand right now to combat the breast cancer enemy.

REFERENCES

1. Fisher B Fisher ER Redmond C Brown A.Tumor nuclear grade, estrogen receptor, and progesterone receptor: their value alone or in combination as indicators of outcome following adjuvant therapy for breast cancer. Breast Cancer Res Treat 1986;7(3):147-60

2. von Rueden DG Wilson RE Intraductal carcinoma of the breast. Surg Gynecol Obstet 1984 Feb; 158(2):105-11

3. Fisher, ER, The Pathologist's Role in the Diagnosis and Treatment of invasive breast cancer, Symposium on breast cancer, Surg Clin Nor Amer 58:4 Aug 1978 705-720

4. Beahrs OH : Staging cancer, Ca-A Can J for Physicians 41:2 March/April 1991

5. Hems G : Epidemiological characteristics of breast cancer in middle and late age. Brit J Cancer 74:226-234 1970

6. Munzarova M Kovarik J Hlavkova J Kolcova V Course of breast cancer disease and ABO blood groups. Biomed Pharmacother 1985; 39(9-10):486-9

7. Olszewski W, darzynkiewwicz A, Rosen P et al: Flowcytometry of breast carcinoma: I Relation of DNA Ploidy level to histology and estrogen receptor. Cancer 48:980-984, 1981

CHAPTER SEVEN

THE BATTLE PLAN—What is the Best Treatment for Breast Cancer Today?

*a*carefully conceived plan of action is the key to success no matter what the occasion. Whether it's Thanksgiving turkey with all the trimmings or the wedding of the year with all the frills, any successful event requires forethought and planning.

Team sports are good examples where planning means winning. All teams study their opponents and map out a plan for winning. They call it the game plan. In football, with all the brute physical contact, I believe, you will agree, it's really a battle plan. It's flexible and the coach can change it on the spot to cope with changing circumstances of the game.

Obviously, the battle plan to control and eradicate disease also continues to change in light of new medical discoveries and innovative technology. Careful planning and attention to the game plan have led to marvelous victories in the medical field; and over the years many dread diseases in this country, such as small pox, measles, and polio, have been controlled or eliminated. Breakthroughs in treating certain cancers, such as childhood leukemia have also been achieved in our time.

In spite of these advances in medical sophistica-

The strategy today in the struggle against breast cancer calls for painstaking development and testing of new anti-cancer weapons. It is now believed to be a systemic disease rather than localized, almost from the very beginning.
• • • • • • •

tion, the battles to conquer major cancers, such as lung, colon, breast, pancreas, and prostate are often tedious with too few victories to record.

In this chapter let's examine how the battle against breast cancer is progressing. Are there any victories we can point to? Are there any victories on the horizon? Let's review the different treatment strategies promulgated by today's experienced clinicians.

———

For a long time we attacked breast cancer like the early football player, sloshing through the mud with the snug helmet and baggy pants, with only a make shift game plan. We were akin to the Roman legions with only spear and shield, waging war on breast cancer by radical, mutilating surgery.

Now, times have changed. Football has become a safer sport with advances in equipment and technique. The basic weapons of war and defense are no longer the Roman spear and shield; and the battle plan to control breast cancer has also changed and continues to evolve.

The strategy today in the struggle against breast cancer calls for painstaking development and testing of new anti-cancer weapons. Many years are spent testing and comparing treatment programs; and when there are variations of many therapies and several combinations of complicated treatment protocols, defining the best therapy is often imprecise.

Nevertheless, we have come some distance in recent decades in changing our general philosophy on how breast cancer should be attacked. It is now believed to be a systemic disease rather than localized, almost from the very beginning. There has also been advances in our knowledge of how the body's natural defenses operate, and how those defense systems can be enhanced.

However, there remains a diminishing residue of personal bias and passion for entrenched ideas that occasionally confuse the issue when defining the optimal plan. Statistics have been used to reflect forgone conclusions. Doctors quoting the same statistics have drawn diametrically opposing conclusions. Someone once said, "There are liars, damn liars, and statistics". Here's an example. A study at the Guy Hospital in London compared the radical mastectomy to local excision and radiation.[1] The five year survival favored the radical mastectomy in Stage II cases and was widely quoted by proponents favoring radical surgery. The *ten year* survival, however, showed no statistical difference and that figure, naturally was quoted by the radiation enthusiasts. Nevertheless, through research and carefully planned clinical trials, and with less emotion and bias, modern weapons required to destroy breast cancer are being forged.

At the turn of the century the battle cry of most surgeons in America was, "Cut out as much as you can". Of course there were dissenters. The French surgeon, Matas, in 1900, Dr. George Crile, Sr., in the 1920's, and Dr. Keynes of England, in the 1930's, were convinced that a lesser surgery was adequate; but their ideas fell on deaf ears.[2] The notion that radical surgery was the only way to control and cure breast cancer was firmly planted in the American surgical dogma; and the vast majority of surgeons followed this dictum in lock-step for the next 75 years.

Radiation to treat breast cancer came on the scene in the 1930's and 1940's. As you might imagine X-ray machines were little more than simple radiation emitters in the early days. The correct radiation dose was unknown and the results were unpredictable and often tragic.

About the same time it was observed that estrogens helped some post-menopausal women and castration prolonged life in a minority of younger women before the menopause. However there was no way to predict who would be helped.

Next came Dr. Huggin's work in the 1950's, demonstrating the value of adrenalectomy and hypophysectomy (removal of the adrenal and pituitary glands).[3] This new battle plan, however, was compromised by significant morbidity and death.

Finally, chemotherapy was introduced in the 1960's with its own set of complications such as hair loss, severe nausea, bone marrow depression and even death. Subsequent combinations of these drugs have been used to the advantage, and some lengthening of life has been reported.

Various investigators pleaded for radiation early in the battle. Others decried radiation in favor of surgery only; and there were many protagonists advocating different forms of surgery and combinations of surgery and radiation. Finally, some proponents spoke of a melding of radiation, chemotherapy, hormones, and surgery. These debates often generated more heat than light.

Even today the battle plan is still being focused and redefined; and I suspect it will continue in a state of flux until various treatments are measured and compared. Trials are going forth, and perhaps in the next ten years the very best treatment will be defined.

Presently, treatment decisions must be designed for the individual woman with the best information available. It is absolutely imperative that physicians who treat breast cancer be aware of new therapies on the horizon that will afford his patient optimum care.

In well over half the breast cancer cases found in black women, cancer has already spread beyond the confines of the breast when the diagnosis is made.

In well over half the breast cancer cases found in black women, cancer has already spread beyond the confines of the breast when the diagnosis is made.[4] It can be detected in the axilla, the lung, the bone and the liver. In early cases, when spread cannot be detected, there remains a twenty percent chance of undetectable metastasis. Surgery and radiation can only hope to control the primary site and local lymph node spread. The body's inherent immune system usually deals effectively with microscopic dissemination. However, immunity can quickly be overwhelmed and the patient rendered unable to deal with a large host of tumor cells. At that point chemotherapy may be helpful but not curative. Chemotherapy should not be used too soon since investigators have shown that drugs used prematurely can impair the immune system to the patient's detriment.

The most recent weapons include the anti-estrogen Tamoxifen and a more precise use of estrogen. These additions to the battle plan will be discussed further in this chapter.

For the reader who is not inclined to know the details in the development of various treatment methods please turn to the segment, THE BATTLE PLAN TODAY, at the end of this chapter. However, for those wanting an overview of how we got to where we are today in treating breast cancer, the following paragraphs should be helpful.

THE HALSTEAD RADICAL MASTECTOMY

In 1894 William Halstead of the Johns Hopkins Medical Center in Baltimore, devised the radical mastectomy: The same operation thousands of surgeons world-wide have performed over the decades.[5]

The nipple and a large segment of skin along with the entire breast and underlying muscle on the chest wall (pectoralis major and pectoralis minor), plus the fat containing lymph nodes of the axilla were excised enbloc, that is altogether, as a single specimen (please refer to Chapter Two).

Emphasis was placed on the enbloc dissection because of the penetration and contiguous spread of these neglected cases that were presented to Dr Halstead at the turn of the century. Halstead believed that cutting through the specimen would possibly spread cancer cells, so he insisted on removing the entire specimen intact. In 1907 he reported in the medical literature his experience with 232 patients.[6]

Dr Halstead found that breast cancers in his patients were often large and bulky and sometimes hidden for years before the patient finally came to surgery. Some of those cancers involved deep penetration into the muscle. Others broke onto the chest wall disrupting the skin. Although these were far advanced neglected cases, Halstead reported that 32.2 percent survived three years and 29.8 percent lived five years or more.[6] These figures of late stage cancer survival compare very well with our results today. Although this was a disfiguring operation it was argued that the cure rate was better than any other procedure available. With improvement of surgical technique and control of infection, survival continued to improved until the 1940's and early 1950's. But from 1950 onward, the cure rate has not substantially improved. The surgery offered today is much less disfiguring, but is no better in effecting a cure than the Halstead operation of 1894.

The Halstead radical mastectomy was the standard battle plan that American surgeons depended upon,

***T**he Halstead radical mastectomy was the standard battle plan that American surgeons depended upon, and all other procedures and treatments introduced since 1894 have invariably been compared to this surgical milestone.*
● ● ● ● ● ● ●

and all other procedures and treatments introduced since 1894 have invariably been compared to this surgical milestone.

Radical mastectomy was found to be fraught with morbidity and complications. Massive swelling of the arm was often encountered when lymphatic vessels and blood vessels were necessarily interrupted. Occasionally infection and nerve injuries were encountered. Stiffness and pain of the shoulder and scaring played havoc with rehabilitation efforts.

In view of these complications and the static cure rate over the past four generations, physicians and patients alike were soon looking for a new battle plan. In the mid-1950's clinicians in Europe and the United States were testing less radical alternatives for dealing with breast cancer. In England and France radiation therapy following limited surgery replaced the standard radical mastectomy as the bulwark of breast cancer control. Their results were good, although not quite as good as the Halstead procedure if cancer had already spread to the regional lymph nodes.

As later work would show, the dose of radiation used in those early European trials was insufficient. With an adjustment of the radiation it was shown that limited surgery with radiation was as good as the Halstead and with less complications. In 1975 Dr. Bernard Pierquin of Paris reported his 15 years experience using radiation following local excision of the tumor to control breast cancer.[7] The results were comparable to radical surgery.

In the 1960's American surgeons such as Dr John Madden in New York, and Dr George Crile, Jr, in Cleveland were openly critical of the Halstead operation for being too extensive.[8,9] Dr Crile became a vigorous advocate of less surgery; and, in fact, he spear-

BREAST CANCER / BLACK WOMAN 119

headed the drive for the limited breast procedures performed today.

Meanwhile investigators in Europe including Dr. Handley of Middlesex Hospital, London, were challenging the sacred cow of radical mastectomy.[10] Data was presented advocating the modified radical mastectomy, a less disfiguring operation with comparable cure rates in early cancers. A new battle plan was in the making. Local control of the cancer, it was argued, could be achieved by removing the cancerous breast and contents of the axilla without compromising survival. Meyer and colleagues in Rockford, Illinois suggested in 1959 and again in 1978 that lesser procedures would have the same cure rate at ten years as the standard Halstead surgery.[11] Then Dr Bernard Fisher, at the University of Pittsburgh, corroborated this finding in the national task force study of alternative breast cancer treatments.[12]

However, other breast specialists in America led by Anglem of Boston and Haagenson of New York, were not persuaded and continued to champion the cause of Halstead's radical approach. They pointed to the so-called Rotter lymph nodes found between the pectoralis major and minor that would be left behind unless the radical surgery was performed. In a blistering rebuttal to Dr Crile, as late as 1974, Dr Anglem defended the radical mastectomy in the strongest terms and emotionally denigrated any lesser procedure.[13] He believed that Crile's data was biased. Anglem was joined by Dr Leis of New York, another Halstead devotee, in noting the high incidence of bilateral disease in young patients. He suggested prophylactic removal of the opposite breast in young cancer patients, in selected cases. Haagenson a respected surgeon and pathologist at Columbia University considered the modified radical mastectomy as a "great leap backward".[14,15]

About the same time, Dr Jerome Urban also of New York, was speaking at surgical gatherings around the country, advocating the radical Halstead and also the super-radical mastectomy if the lesion was located in the medial half of the breast.[16] He had reported his work in 1952 but had few takers at that time. The super-radical in addition to the standard radical, consisted of removing the medial second, third and fourth ribs, along with the underlying lymph nodes. Urban claimed little increase in operating time and no significant morbidity. His statistics indicated an increased local recurrence if the super-radical was not done for cancer located in the medial half of the breast; however, he could not claim increased survival at five and ten years. Very few surgeons followed his lead; and, apparently, no one could duplicate his results. Also the super-radical was out of step with the times.

American women were, by this time, demanding a more conservative approach and a greater voice in determining their treatment. Several investigators had shown that survival was not dependent on the location of the lesion in the breast. With increasing knowledge of the biology of the disease and improved weapons of chemotherapy and radiation available, there is no longer, in my opinion, any further need to debate the utility of the super-radical procedure, or even, for that matter, the Halstead radical mastectomy.

THE MODIFIED RADICAL MASTECTOMY

The most frequent operation for breast cancer performed today in the United States is the modified

Limited surgery with radiation was as good as the Halstead radical surgery, and with less complications.

radical mastectomy or so-called total mastectomy with axillary dissection. In this operation the cancerous breast is entirely removed including the nipple and a limited amount of skin. The muscles under the breast are preserved. The axillary contents are removed enbloc along with the breast, or through a separate axillary incision.

Dr Donald Patey, reporting in the British Journal of Cancer in 1967, described 156 cases operated in this manner between 1930 and 1943.[17] He removed the pectoralis minor muscle and spared the large pectoralis major. This has been modified and today both muscles are left in place. Patey used the term total mastectomy with axillary dissection. The results were good and comparable to the radical mastectomy, but there was little response in those years from surgeons on this side of the Atlantic. Neither Patey nor Handley of London was a match for Halstead's disciples. Perhaps Americans were a bit provincial and favored the American way of doing things. The British surgeons did not claim that their operation held out any improvement in cure rate, only that it was less disfiguring. In the pre-1960's disfigurement was not of major concern to the American surgeons. The destruction of cancer was the only goal.

Nevertheless, over the ensuing 20 years a growing number of American doctors began to boldly support

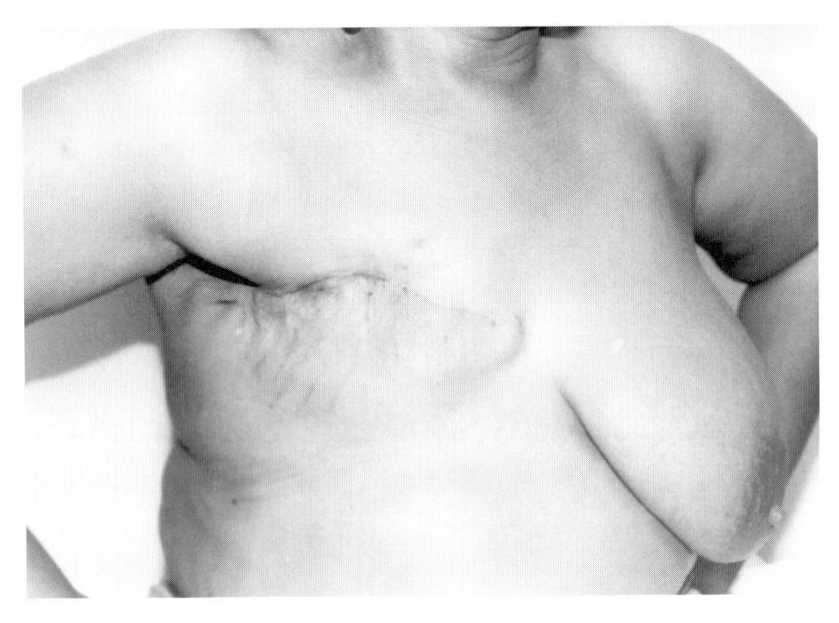

Fig. 7-1
MODIFIED RADICAL MASTECTOMY. This is the most common surgery done for breast cancer in the United States. The entire breast has been removed, but there is a thick layer of fat and the underlying muscles have been left intact. This allows for a more satisfactory appearance of the chest wall and facilitates the use of the brassiere prosthesis. If plastic surgery is contemplated, the plastic surgeon is able to utilize the tissue to advantage.

the notion of less surgery in early cases and avoiding mutilation without compromising the chance of cure. No doubt American medicine was responding to an outcry against too many tonsillectomies, too many hysterectomies and breast surgery that was too radical.

In the early 1970s Dr Delarue of Toronto General Hospital, found that modified radical mastectomy resulted in a comparable number of cures as the standard Halstead radical surgery, provided the muscle was not invaded and the apical nodes not involved.[18]

In 1977 Dr Bernard Fisher, in Pittsburgh, made his first report of clinical trials from 68 medical centers comparing radical mastectomy to total mastectomy with radiation.[19] After exhaustive analysis of the data, Dr Fisher and his colleagues concluded that there was no real difference regarding survival between radical and modified radical surgery plus radiation.

In Dr Fisher's second report a look at the ten year results were available.[20] Again the data continued to support the notion that the radical mastectomy was not required in Stage I and II disease when the muscle was not grossly involved. Many others have found no difference in long term survivorship between radical and modified radical surgery, coupled with radiation and chemotherapy.

PARTIAL MASTECTOMY

This surgical procedure championed by Crile and others since 1955 consists of excising a generous section of breast with the tumor along with the lower group of axillary nodes. The cure rate overall is not as good as the Halstead. In selected cases, however, according to Crile, the results are indeed comparable to radical surgery, and the contour of the breast is preserved. This means the lesion must be small and located in an outer quadrant and not fixed to the skin or underlying muscle. Few black patients present with these early lesions and few blacks are amenable to this ultra-limited surgery.

If the cancer is found early and is small and localized, Crile found that this limited surgery is every bit as curative as the Halstead radical surgery. Strict guidelines were laid down. The cancer should be small, of a certain size, and other hazardous diseases should not be present. Advanced age was another adverse criteria. Dr Crile reported 57 patients treated between 1955 and 1964 with a 67 percent five year overall control. Later results improved when this limited surgery was combined with radiation.[21]

Dr Umberto Veronesi of Milan, Italy, reported his experience using a quadrectomy (removal of the quadrant of breast bearing the cancer) with axillary dissection and radiation.[22] His data over a fifteen year period was equal to the Halstead radical surgery without the mutilation, thus corroborating the work of Crile and others.

LUMPECTOMY AND RADIATION

Since the early 1960's doctors in England and France have used excision of the cancer with only a small rim of normal tissue combined with radiation as their primary weapon. In over 95 percent of the cases the contour of the breast is preserved and they believe that their cure rate is as good as the radical Halstead. There is no serious doubt that radiation in adequate dosage is able to kill micro-foci of breast cancer cells.

Few black patients present with these early lesions and few blacks are amenable to this ultra-limited surgery.

> *Conservative surgery with radiation and even radiation alone in small cancers is widely available. Several States, including Massachusetts, California and Wisconsin have mandated that physicians inform patients with breast cancer of alternative treatments.*

Radiation following lumpectomy is vital since it is known that many cancers are multi-centric in origin. In short, the major lump may be removed but residual microscopic tumor may be left in the remaining breast. A study at Memorial Hospital in New York showed that microscopic cancers that were unsuspected were found in 26 percent of breasts removed for a dominant cancerous lump. It is not certain that these microscopic foci of cancer would ever become clinically important. In a study of women over seventy who died of causes other than breast cancer, microscopic cancer of the breast was found at a rate nineteen times expected for that age group. Microscopic thyroid cancers are also noted that never cause clinical cancer disease and 40 percent of elderly men have microscopic prostatic cancer that never becomes manifest.

Conservative surgery with radiation and even radiation alone in small cancers is widely available. Several States, including Massachusetts, California and Wisconsin have mandated that physicians inform patients with breast cancer of alternative treatments. Long trials using radiation and limited, breast-saving surgery have been concluded by Dr Bernard Fisher; and the results in 1985 indicate that in early breast cancers limited surgery, sparing the breast, with radiation can be as curative as more extensive surgery.[23]

The protocol usually runs like this: The tumor is excised through a small incision and through a separate incision the lower lymph nodes from the axilla are removed. If there is cancer in those lymph nodes, and the patient has not gone through menopause, she is also given chemotherapy or the anti-estrogen, Tamoxifen. Next, external beam orthovoltage, using either cobalt or the linear accelerator, is directed over the entire breast to remove any micro-foci of cancer. If the primary cancer is over 2.5 centimeters, Irridium can be implanted at the operative site to boost the radiation dose. External beam radiation is also directed over regional lymph nodes in the axillary, supraclavicular and internal mammary sites as well. A total of 5000 rads per week for 5 weeks controls microscopic invasive cancer in over 90 percent of cases. If axillary nodes are clinically enlarged, the dosage is boosted by 1000 to 2000 rads in that particular area.

In 1977 several medical centers in the U.S. reported results of a combined trial using radiation and local excision. The breast was spared and 75 percent of the patients had an excellent cosmetic result. Moreover they showed a five year survival of 91 percent in Stage I and 75 percent survival in Stage II patients. These figures compare very well with patients undergoing radical mastectomy.[24] In 1982 the French provided proof that at fifteen years the survival of patients with the lesser procedure and radiation were as good as the radical mastectomy.

At the Joint Center for Radiation Therapy, a prestigious cancer treatment center in Boston, Dr Martin Levene and others are treating breast cancer by local excision of the tumor, leaving the remainder of the breast intact, followed by local and regional radiation.[25] Radiation is administered by external beam to the axilla, and Irridium is implanted at the site of the tumor excision if total removal is in doubt. In Stage I they report a 91 percent disease-free state at 5 years, and for Stage II a 60 percent disease-free state. Even Stage III showed a 26 percent survival at five years.

There remain very few pockets of skepticism among physicians. Some radiotherapists will accept only

Stage I or Stage II women that are highly motivated to forego mastectomy. Some women faced with cancer continue to find greater security with mastectomy than radiation treatment; and there are surgeons who will not suggest to their patients a lumpectomy over a mastectomy even though it is available for those meeting certain criteria. It's up to the patient to question their doctor whether or not their case falls within the guidelines for lumpectomy and radiation.

Complications associated with radiation must be carefully considered. The patient routinely will find skin irritation, difficulty in swallowing and tracheitis (inflammation of the wind pipe), esophagitis, and rarely rib fracture.

The immune system may be impaired, thus making the patient more susceptible to pneumonia and other infection. Serious complications, however, are unusual and should not dissuade the patient or the attentive radiotherapist. In a report from Harvard, 88 percent of a group of patients treated with radiation and followed up to seven years judged the cosmetic result as excellent or good.[26] The texture of the breast may show increased firmness and there may be a slight decrease in breast size. Often it is difficult to tell on casual inspection which breast was treated.

Despite occasional setbacks the trend towards a more prominent role for radiation and conservative surgery has altered the battle plan in the breast cancer war. In Stages I and II, the radical Halstead is a thing of the past. Only in Stage III with bulky tumors, with fixation against the chest wall, would some surgeons perform a radical mastectomy. Dr Guy Robbins, former chief of the Breast Service of Memorial Hospital, New York, and other prominent surgeons, believe this is an indication for the Halstead radical

It's up to the patient to question their doctor whether or not their case falls within the guidelines for lumpectomy and radiation.

mastectomy. On the other hand, Crile and Fisher, equally astute, believe that there is no place for radical breast surgery today; and indeed, the data seem to support the view of conservatism.

The Blue Shield Plan of New Jersey reported that medical claims for radical mastectomy dropped 75 percent between 1974 and 1982 and the modified radical increased by 50 percent. All forms of breast amputation have continued to decrease in spite of the increased incidence of breast cancer. In the 1990's radical mastectomy is rarely done and any such procedure draws the immediate attention of peer review.

HORMONES AND CHEMOTHERAPY

As new potent weapons are developed, strategy and tactics will obviously change. We now find in our arsenal a growing array of drugs and hormones. These armaments are now ready and available to assail the metastatic cancer that is often in transit when the gross breast cancer is first discovered. Consequently, many clinicians believe that all Stage III women should have chemotherapy and Stage II patients as well, if the axillary nodes are enlarged. Preliminary reports are suggesting that the outlook is improved, and perhaps one can be cured by adding chemotherapy (CMF and Tamoxifen) immediately at the time of limited surgery. This data has been developed by Fisher, and if it continues to hold up in the 1990s as it seems to be, it will represent the greatest triumph against breast cancer in the past fifty years.[27]

From 1945 to 1960 hormone therapy (estrogen, testosterone, and castration) was the major weapon in the control of metastatic breast cancer. But the physician had no way to predict the response and it was

All forms of breast amputation have continued to decrease in spite of the increased incidence of breast cancer. In the 1990's radical mastectomy is rarely done and any such procedure draws the immediate attention of peer review.

Combination chemotherapy most often used in the U.S. include CMF (cyclophosphamide, methyltrexate, 5-florouracil). In 1993, CMF remains the standard chemotherapy for breast cancer.
• • • • • • •

actually a shot in the dark proposition. A few of the patients that did have a remission could expect additional control with removal of the adrenal glands or hypophysectomy. However, the morbidity and mortality of these operations was formidable.

Between 1960 and 1970 single agent chemotherapy was in vogue, almost completely replacing hormone treatment. These weapons led to excess morbidity and mortality as dosage requirements and tolerance of the patient were not completely elucidated.

The years 1970 to 1975 saw the emergence of combination chemotherapy (the use of more than one anti-cancer drug) with improved longevity. The combination most often used in the U.S. then and now include CMF (cyclophosphamide, methyltrexate, 5-florouracil), and CAF (cyclophosphamide, Adriamycin, 5-florouracil) for advanced cancer. L-pam (l-phenylalanine mustard) plus 5-florouracil has found some success in Stage II premenopausal patients at the time of limited surgery.

In 1993, CMF remains the standard chemotherapy for breast cancer. The drugs are combined with Tamoxifen in all Stage II patients of all ages that are estrogen receptor positive (ER-positive).

ESTROGEN RECEPTOR AND PROGESTERONE RECEPTOR

In the early 1970's researchers at the University of Chicago and elsewhere gave us the Estrogen Receptor Theory. It has proved to be a device that has allowed us to direct hormone and chemotherapy to patients that may respond. Here's the way it operates. First, it was noted by Glascock in 1959, that if an estrogen was labeled so you could follow it through the body; and it was injected into a laboratory animal, it would congregate in the ovary and breast tissue. It was further found that if the animal was first given breast cancer and then injected with estrogen, the hormone had a propensity to be taken up by some of the cancer cells. As it turned out, a protein inside the cancer cell was necessary to receive the incoming estrogen. This protein was named estrogen receptor (ER). However, in many cancer cells it was not present and, consequently, the estrogen was not taken up by those malignant cells.

By the early 1970's investigators had shown that some 60 to 70 percent of the human breast cancer cells contained estrogen receptor protein. This suggested that the cancer was estrogen dependent, and in the premenopausal patient if estrogen was denied the body by removing the ovaries, a remission of cancer was theoretically possible. As it turned out, however, only about half of these women were helped by removal of the ovaries. Further study revealed that it wasn't an all or nothing situation. Cancer cells had different levels of estrogen receptor. When the level was quantified, then one noted that if a patient's cancer cells had a very high level of ER, response to hormonal manipulation would be 65 percent. If the ER was absent or very low, the response was only six percent.

Building on these observations, it was soon discovered that progesterone receptors also occurred in breast cancer cells. Progesterone, another ovarian hormone, when placed in proximity to cancer cells, would enter those that contained a progesterone receptor. One could correlate the likelihood of hormone response to the presence of progesterone receptor. Patients that have both ER and progesterone receptor positive cancer cells have about an 80 percent favorable response to hormonal and chemotherapy treatment.[28]

Consequently, a check of the ER level and progesterone receptor level of cancer removed at surgery is a must, since only an average or high titer of receptor level would pose a rational basis to prescribe castration, adrenalectomy, hypophysectomy or chemotherapy. Should the premenopausal black woman with metastatic breast cancer be ER positive of high titer, she would have a 65 percent chance of responding to removal of the ovaries by surgery or radiation. This would control the metastasis for about 12 months—sometimes for several years. On the other hand, postmenopausal black women who are ER positive respond to the administration of estrogen in 65 percent of cases. Just how this change in hormone status operates in pre and postmenopausal women remains unknown.

The ER positive women who are fortunate enough to respond to the initial hormonal manipulation may find a second remission following adrenalectomy or hypophysectomy. Fifty-five percent of premenopausal and 75 percent of post menopausal ER positive women will respond to these second treatments. With recent advances in surgical technique, most physicians favor the trans-sphenoid hypophysectomy over the adrenalectomy. Through these measures the cancer enemy can be held at bay for another 6 to 18 months. In a few cases remission may last many years.

TAMOXIFEN

Since 1976, a new battery of cancer-fighting tools called antiestrogens have been brought to the struggle.

The most common agent in this class is Tamoxifen. By 1992 it had been fairly well tested by Dr Fisher and his colleagues, and a definite place in the treatment protocol was outlined.[29] Essentially tamoxifen blocks the action of estrogen which is thought to perpetuate cancer. If a patient has a very high level of ER positivity she will almost always respond to Tamoxifen. There are almost no side effects and the drug seems to be safe with no real contraindications. It can be combined with standard chemotherapy and it has been shown to give added benefit especially in those patients over 50 years of age. This antiestrogen is being used more and more in cases that formerly were treated with hypophysectomy or adrenalectomy.

IMMUNOTHERAPY

The immune system is that set of mechanisms incorporated in the body to help defend itself against invading bacteria, viruses, foreign matter, and cancer. One gains immunity when the body recognizes a particle, a substance, or a cancer as a foreign intruder called antigen. The body, through an elaborate system in response to the antigen, produces antibodies designed to resist and destroy the invader. The antibody formed is sometimes very specific and will attack only the antigen that caused the specific antibody to form.

Other antibodies are not specific and will go about destroying all foreign substances. For example, it has been found that the bacterium C. parvum will stimulate the production of antibodies against not only this particular bacterium but also against certain cancer cells as well. It has been shown that patients receiving chemotherapy survive much longer when this antigen, C. parvum, is incorporated in the protocol.

In spite of the appeal of immunotherapy the results have not been consistent. It has not been a reliable asset in treating early or late stages of breast cancer. Immunotherapy, remains experimental.
● ● ● ● ● ● ●

In another example, it is known that Bacillus Calumette Guerre (BCG) serves as an antigen against Mycobacteria bovis. It stimulates antibody formation not only against M. bovis but also against M. tuberculosis, thus immunizing against tuberculosis. For some unknown reason it also can offer some protection against certain cancers. In Stage II breast cancer investigators using BCG noted only a 5 percent relapse rate compared to a 40 percent relapse rate in patients not using BCG. Levamisole, another antigen, with non-specificity in antibody formation is also being tried in the search for cancer immunotherapy.

In spite of the appeal of immunotherapy the results have not been consistent. There's still too many unanswered questions, and overall, it has not been a reliable asset in treating early or late stages of breast cancer. Consequently, immunotherapy, that is, using the immune system to control cancer, remains experimental and only controlled trials are being conducted. It is not available for most patients. Several protocols combining immunotherapy with chemotherapy, radiation and/or surgery are being suggested. It remains to be seen whether or not a protocol of hormones and immunotherapy combined will find a place in preventive or palliative care.

THE BATTLE PLAN TODAY

In reviewing the overall strategy developed since 1970, our first line of defense and our most potent weapon remains surgery.

In the 1990s either the modified radical mastectomy, or lumpectomy plus radiation with separate removal of axillary nodes for Stages I and II, would be appropriate.

The majority of women with Stage I or II are cured today with the weapons we have at hand.

• • • • • • •

The Halstead radical mastectomy for Stage III cancer is rarely advocated in most major centers; and most surgeons, I suspect, will not find the need for radical surgery in any circumstance.

If there is local spread to lymph nodes as in Stage II, then chemotherapy and Tamoxifen would be in order in the estrogen-receptor positive **pre-menopausal** patient. Some doctors would use these agents prophylactically even if there are no obvious metastases. In the estrogen receptor negative patient, Tamoxifen and chemotherapy will be much less effective.

In the **postmenopausal** patient, under similar conditions, similar surgery and radiation, followed by Tamoxifen is the standard care today for the estrogen receptor positive patient. Chemotherapy is usually withheld in estrogen negative patients unless there is clear evidence of metastasis. This is because the side effects of chemotherapy cannot be justified in the face of the known poor therapeutic results of chemotherapy in older women.

The combination of chemotherapy, Tamoxifen, and palliative radiotherapy is usually prescribed in Stage IV breast cancer.

There continues to be lingering skepticism with regards sparing the breast and combining very limited surgery with radiation or chemotherapy. The data seem impressive and trials continue. I expect the use of limited surgery and radiation will continue to increase in the United States and eventually become the treatment of choice in this country as it is in Europe.

Some physicians prefer chemotherapy over radiation because radiation only kills the local cancer. Chemotherapy at the time of limited surgery kills not only local cancer but metastatic foci as well. There is mounting evidence in premenopausal women that early chemotherapy at the time of surgery is beneficial.

The second line of defense becomes a holding action. This applies to patients who've had a relapse following initial control of their disease. In this phase we are concerned with prolonging life and enhancing the quality of life. The weapons used depend on the estrogen-receptor (ER) status of the cancer. If it is positive, then a majority of patients will respond to hormonal manipulation. For the ER negative patients we must retreat immediately to chemotherapy. The ER positive women who respond to removal of the ovaries or hormonal therapy, will often have a second remission following adrenalectomy or hypophysectomy. However, because of attendant morbidity and complications, many physicians will forego these procedures and go directly to Tamoxifen, the anti-estrogen that has been effective in both pre-and post-menopausal women. Using these treatments life can be prolonged for many months or several years.

The majority of women with Stage I or II are cured today with the weapons we have at hand, but the ultimate victory in more advanced cases may require more sophisticated intervention. In the coming decades, artillery now on the drawing boards will be added to the battle plan. New combinations of surgery, chemotherapy, radiotherapy, hormonal therapy, immunotherapy and even hyperthermia (heating the cancer or the whole body) may well be part of tomorrow's arsenal to combat cancer.

Interferon, a substance produced by the body in response to viral invasion and other attacks, appears to enhance the immune system. It also appears to stimulate anti-tumor killer cells to destroy cancer. In one study 25 percent of patients with advanced breast

> *Patients who've had a relapse following initial control of their disease—we are concerned with prolonging life and enhancing the quality of life.*

cancer found remission with interferon treatment. However, there have been unacceptable side effects, and supply and purity have also been a problem.

It has been found that cancer cells require enormous amounts of cysteine. In the laboratory animal, if this essential amino acid is removed from the body, cancer cells die; however, before it proves fatal to the animal, cysteine can be replaced. Hence, the cancer cells are eliminated and the animal is cured.

———

With these examples of ingenuity and innovation it's only a matter of time before we witness the final assault on breast cancer. Until that time the key to the battle plan will continue to be prompt discovery, mainly by women who are aware and alert, and intervention by doctors who remain on the cutting edge of the struggle against this dread disease.

Having followed the battle plan, the next step is to get on with life—day by day.

REFERENCES

1. Atkins H, Hayward JL, Klugman DJ: Treatment of early breast cancer: a report after ten years of a clinical trial. Brit Med J 423-429 May 20 1972

2. Keynes G: Conservative treatment of cancer of the breast. Br Med J 1937; 2:643-647

3. Huggins C, Dao T: Characteristics of adrenal dependent mammary cancer. Ann Surg 140:497 1954

4. Coates RJ Bransfield DD Wesley M Hankey B Eley JW Greenberg RS. Flanders D Hunter CP Edwards BK Forman M et al: Differences between black and white women with breast cancer in time from symptom recognition to medical consultation. Black/White Cancer Survival Study Group. J Natl Cancer Inst (1992 Jun 17) 84(12):938-50

5. Halstead WS: The results of operations for the cure of cancer of the breast performed at Johns Hopkins hospital from June 1889 to January 1894. Ann Surg 20:497-550 1894

6. Halstead WS: The results of radical operations for the cure of cancer of the breast. Ann Surg 46:1 1907

7. Pierquin B, Baillet F, Wilson JF: Radiation therapy in the management of primary breast cancer. Am J Roentgenol Rad Ther Nucl Med 127:645-648 1976

8. Crile G Jr: Simplified treatment of cancer of the breast: early results of a clinical study. Ann Surg 1961 153:745

9. Madden JL, Modified radical mastectomy: SG&O 121:6 1221-1230 Dec 1965

10. Handley RS, Thackray AC:Conservative radical mastectomy (Patey's operation). Ann Surg 880-882 Dec 1969

11. Meyer AC, Smith SS, Potter M: Carcinoma of the breast a clinical study. Arch Surg 113:364-368 April 1978

12. Fisher B: Breast cancer management: Alternatives to radical mastectomy. N Engl J Med 301:326-329, 1979

13. Anglem TJ: Management of breast cancer: radical mastectomy. JAMA 230:1 99-105 Oct 7 1974

14. Haagensen CD: A great leap backward in the treatment of carcinoma of the breast. JAMA 224:1181-1183

15. Haagensen CD, Bodian C: A personal experience with Halsted's radial mastectomy. Amer Journ Surg 199:2 143-150 Feb 1984

16. Urban JA, Baker HW: Radical mastectomy in continuity with enbloc resection of the internal mammary lymph-node chain. Cancer 5:5 992-1008 Sept 1952

17. Patey D: A review of 146 cases of carcinoma of the breast operated on between 1930 and 1943. Br J Cancer 21:260-269,1967

18. Delarue NC, Anderson WD, Starr J: Modified radical mastectomy in the individualized treatment of breast carcinoma. SG&O 79-88 July 1969

19. Fisher B, Montague E, Redmond C, et al: Comparison of radical mastectomy with alternative treatments for primary breast cancer: A first report of results from a prospective randomized clinical trial, Cancer 39:2827 1977

20. Fisher B, Wolmark N: Limited surgical management for primary breast cancer: a commentary on the NSABP report. World J Surg 9:5 682-691 Oct 1985

21. Crile G JR, Esselstyn CV Jr, Hermann RE, et al: Partial mastectomy for carcinoma of the breast. SG&O 136:929-933 1973

22. Veronesi U, Saccozzi R, Del Vecchio M, et al: Comparing radical mastectomy with quadrantectomy, axillary dissection and radotherapy in patients with small cancers of the breast. NEJM 305:6-11 July 2 1981

23. Fisher B, Wolmark N, Fisher ER, et al: Lumpectomy and axillary dissection for breast cancer: surgical, pathological and radiation considerations. Wor J Surg 9:692-698 1985.

24. Fisher, B Montague E Redmond C et al: Comparison of radical mastectomy with alternative treatments for primary breast cancer: A first report of results from a prospective randomized clinical trial. Cancer 39:2827 1977

25. Levene MB, Harris Jr, Hellman S: Treatment of carcinoma of the breast by radiation therapy. Cancer 39:6 2840-2845 June Suppl 1977

26. Rose MA, Olivotto I Cady B et al: Conservative surgery and radiation therapy for early breast cancer: Long-term cosmetic results. Arch Surg 124:153-157 1989

27. Fisher B, Redmond C, Brown A, et al: Treatment of primary breast cancer with chemotherapy and tamoxifen. NeJM 305:1 1-11 July 2, 1981

28. Block GE, Ellis RS, Desombre E, et al: Correlation of estrophilin content of primary mammary cancer to eventual endocrine treatment. Ann Surg 188:3 372-376 Sept 1978

29. Fisher B: A biological perspective of breast cancer: contributions of the national surgical adjuvant breast and bowel project clinical trials Ca-Can J for Physicians 41:2 March/April 1991

Even though Estrogens may be efficacious in treating menopausal symptoms and may reduce heart attacks by up to 50% and alleviate osteoporosis, there may be deleterious effects for women treated for breast cancer.

Hindle WH, Estrogen therapy and breast cancer...Breast Diseases 3:4 1992

CHAPTER EIGHT

LIGHTS, CAMERA, ACTION!
The Show Must Go On

Some years ago I made a house call on Abby Lincoln. Abby was in town for a singing engagement at one of the clubs, but the cool San Francisco weather had gotten to her. She had the flu.

In those days, doctors made house calls all the time; so when she called I responded: "Sure", I'll be right over. Where are you staying?" I scratched the hotel room in my notebook and in about thirty minutes or so I was greeted at the door by an obviously ill lady, who waved me in while caught up in a fit of cough and sputter. She apparently spied my bag and guessed I was the doctor.

"You're Doctor Johnson, right?", she asked with a gravelly voice while stumbling towards the bed. "Thanks for coming. I feel awful."

Her voice was heavy and hoarse. Her eyes were red and running and her nose was swollen and congested. Every few minutes she coughed heavily, covering her face with Kleenix.

"Yes, Miss Lincoln. Let me help you back to bed. How long have you been sick?"

"Oh, just call me Abby. I've been coughing all day."

"Alright—Abby". Hmmmm, I thought, as I began the examination.

Blood pressure is fine. Heart normal. Ear drums okay. Wow! Throat red. Lungs congested. Temperature elevated.

Her eyes looked at me questioning. "Just a bad cold, right?"

"For real", I said. "Looks like bronchitis on the way to pneumonia. You need bed rest and medication. In a few days I think you'll be okay. For now you'll have to cancel your engagement and stay put. I don't think you're used to this San Francisco fog." I tried to smile.

She looked at me gloomily. " Doctor it's only seven o'clock. My first show is at ten. Can't you give me some antibiotics or something? The show's got to go on!"

I gave her an injection of antibiotic and three prescriptions. I admired her zeal and drive; however performing was out of the question.

"Did you hear me, Doctor. I've got to sing tonight. I've just got to."

"Sure I understand. But if you're not up to it, just get your medicine, stay in bed, and rest."

A few pleasantries and I was gone. In my mind I knew there was no way Abby would sing that night. No way.

I have been told, and do in part believe, that through rain and snow, through flood and fire, the **mail** must go through. I suppose I accepted that dictum. But did the **show really** have to go on? Even in spite of illness. Was *the show* in the same category as the mail?

Later that night I happened to drop by the club where Abby was supposed to sing. The jazz combo had been playing to rave revues. And I thought I'd take a little R and R, and check them out. Plus I knew the club owner and I had this bit of private knowledge that Miss Lincoln was too sick to come in. I might share that info with the owner or maybe I wouldn't. By the time I got to the club the lights were dimming and the spotlight came on like a shaft of bright through the haze. An ebony rotund balding gentleman in formal attire was making an announcement. I caught the gist through the crowd noise as I made my way in. "Ladies and gentlemen...what you've been waiting for....Miss Abby Lincoln!"

What is this! I don't believe it. But seeing was believing. The spotlight shot to the edge of the platform and it *was* Abby Lincoln. The light caught her smile—sparkling and provocative. Her movements were crisp and animated; her eyes danced and twinkled as the spot light captured the toss of her head and the rhythm in her step. She wore a frilly blouse and cigarette pants with spike heels. Transformed. Stepping high. And she could dance **and** sing. She cleared her throat a couple of times; but there were no excuses about not feeling up to par. The crowd loved her and she loved the crowd. The jazz band was energizing. I mean Abby worked the house and just did her thing for the next 30 minutes. Everybody clapped, stomped, and bellowed; and I just sat back in disbelief. It was unreal. What is this business about the 'show must go on?' Is there something to it after all?

I **knew** Abby had to be feeling bad that night. How did she pull it off? It had to be sheer will power—mind over matter. Dedicated to the performance. Unwilling to let her audience or herself down. I could hear a little rasp in her voice and perhaps her eyes were a little red. But who cared. The lady took care of business. And only her doctor knew.

Now that I think about it, I've seen something like that in my own family and you've seen it too. Struggling against one adversity after another for a greater purpose. In fact we see it around us all the time. Folks

> *There always seems to be someone a little worse off who is surviving and overcoming some handicap.*
> • • • • • • •

working long hours in spite of pain. Old women standing on arthritic knees cooking and cleaning house for little more than nothing—maybe bringing home a covered dish of leftovers—but still trying to keep family together. They are all part of the notion that the 'show must go on'.

Even after serious illness such as breast cancer or whatever foul circumstance that should befall, life must still go on. Doctors and nurses, with all of their skill, are important; but they play only supportive roles. If there is support from family and friends, so much the better. But when all is said and done, it is you the patient, the woman, who must rise up, take center stage and face tomorrow. This is your life.

You might say, 'How is this possible? This is not the flu or arthritis! I've just lost my breast and I still may not be cured!'

Well it is possible. I've seen others overcome, and so can you. Here's how to get started. It's the same formula you use when facing any calamity or severe test. First of all, focus carefully on whatever blessings and good fortune you **do** have. Without even thinking very hard you'll begin to realize first one blessing after another. There always seems to be someone a little worse off who is surviving and overcoming some handicap. You'll discover you can be truly thankful for whatever you have, great or small. Then, start praying on a regular basis for courage and strength—and faith—and then act!

Go into action by directing your mind on what to think. My father used to tell me, 'Think big and you'll be big. Think small and you'll be small'. You still have free will, so think good thoughts, do good deeds, control your actions, even your tone of voice as you relate to your family and friends. Even politeness towards casual acquaintances, strangers and even bill collectors will bring a sense of inner peace. The more sunshine you share with others, the more light and warmth will be reflected towards you. And this will nurture **your** life and your survival.

Remember the entertainer, Lola Falana? When faced with a life threatening illness, she remarked, "I'm not cured, but I'm healed." In other words she was saying, "I've come to terms with my life. God is always good and He will be with me no matter what happens."

If you want to be happy, act happy. If you want to be strong, then act strong. Always search for the best part of any circumstance. You'll find that if you act enthusiastic, you will actually become enthusiastic. And those supporting players around you will reflect your attitude and add to your strength and fortitude.

No, you're not superwoman by any means and there are sure to be moments of despair. However, you have a mind with the ability to direct and channel your thoughts! You can compel the mind to think positively, or allow it to drift negatively. Just try it. The mind is the most important part of the body. All other parts serve to keep it functioning. If you were paralyzed from the neck down, you could still be creative. Certainly you can be creative and fulfilled without an arm or a leg, or a breast. Even without the ability to see, one can be productive and creative. Set your thoughts into action, positive action! Never forget that you are the star of the show, and the show must go on, no matter if you've been completely cured or the cord of life has simply been lengthened for a season.

Adjustment following breast cancer treatment means not only physical recovery, but emotional healing as well. Too often, it means learning to live with incurable disease. You **must** minimize the brooding and self-pity. Read books of inspiration. Read of people who've overcome obstacles. Read Psalms and Job, Ecclesiastes and Proverbs. Read about Jesus and Paul. I guarantee you will find power hidden deep inside that you didn't know existed. Read the bible with the purpose of inspiration. This is a time in life for reflection and re-evaluation, a time to set new goals. A time for the mind to go into action.

Once you thank God for what you **do** have, you automatically turn a switch in the mind from negative despair to positive hope. It works for everyone. And once you're on the road to a positive frame of mind, you're ready for rehabilitation and moving on to new pursuits.

REACH TO RECOVERY

The Reach to Recovery Program of the American Cancer Society has given incalculable assistance in the emotional readjustment of the post-mastectomy patient. This is a program of volunteers who visit mastectomy patients several days after surgery with helpful comments and answers to those 'woman to woman' questions.

All volunteers have had the same operation and are matched as nearly as possible with the patient's ethnic background, age, education and economic status.

In 1976 the Reach to Recovery launched their "Man to Man" program in which a husband of a post-mastectomy patient was available to speak by phone on issues that were not strictly medical. This program was designed to allow husbands whose wives were recently operated, to talk with men who had been through the same experience.

Post-mastectomy volunteers give encouragement as no other group can, for they are living proof of what the patient can attain.
• • • • • • •

The idea of one woman with a mastectomy reaching out to lend emotional support to another who had just undergone similar surgery was put forth by Mrs. Teresa Lasser in 1952 following her own mastectomy. She saw the special need for one woman to reach out to another in such a time of stress. In 1969 the American Cancer Society adopted Mrs. Lasser's program and over the years more than a million women have been helped. Volunteers bring helpful pamphlets and brochures. They demonstrate exercises and often provide a temporary prosthesis to be worn home.

Post-mastectomy volunteers give encouragement as no other group can, for they are living proof of what the patient can attain. The Reach to Recovery volunteer can relate her own moment of depression and personal difficulties. Personal vignettes and suggestions for overcoming barriers can be discussed. The volunteer can encourage the patient to exercise and warn against shoulder stiffness. Obviously these volunteers must be carefully selected and trained. They are well groomed, bright and out-going. Ordinarily no more than three hospital visits are made, and only with the approval of the attending physician. In their own unique way they tell the patient, "You are the show and the show must go on".

REHABILITATION AND COMPLICATIONS

Even before treatment is scheduled, the physician is expected to discuss and explain in some detail the type of treatment (surgery, radiation or chemotherapy) he believes is preferable in any particular case. If you or a loved one are being counselled, be sure you do not feel rushed and that all questions are answered to your satisfaction. If surgery is the option, inquire about radiation. If radiation is suggested be certain that all the surgical options are fully aired. A family member, perhaps a daughter or husband, or a trusted friend should be with you to help with the questions since it is often difficult to remember everything you wish to ask. So while you're thinking, your husband or son can join the discussion. If a biopsy has been done, this is the time to discuss the results and implications for prognosis. In these preliminary talks you also want to know the anticipated problems and complications to be faced while recuperating.

For example, one may expect some tightness over the chest wall if a mastectomy has been performed. Deep breathing exercises to inflate the compressed lung are important. Occasionally a chronic cough develops. This is a good time for smokers to stop smoking. Perhaps the doctor can suggest helpful hints to stop smoking.

There may also be arm swelling and shoulder stiffness in many patients. Early swelling may be due to interruption of the lymph channels that serve the arm, or infection at the operative site. Significant swelling is usually temporary and with early physical therapy it generally subsides. For women who have had extensive axillary dissection, arm swelling is serious and requires vigorous sustained treatment including an elastic arm sleeve and antibiotics in addition to physical therapy.

Fig. 8-1
Arm Swelling following mastectomy. This condition is noted frequently after modified radical surgery, but it is usually temporary and subsides with time. Occasionally it persists to some extent and rarely it can be incapacitating.

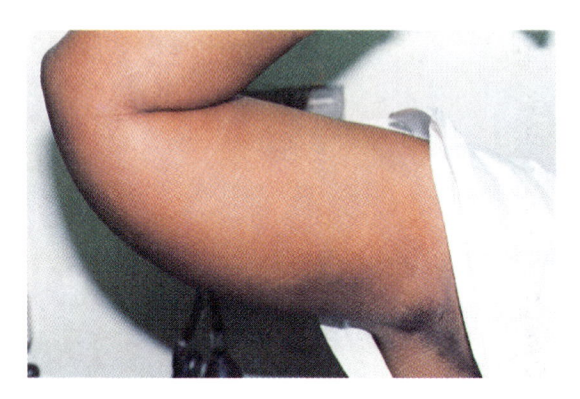

If surgery is the option, inquire about radiation. If radiation is suggested be certain that all the surgical options are fully aired.
● ● ● ● ●

In a small fraction of patients the swelling becomes incapacitating. If neglected the arm can swell three to five times that of the normal arm and become a useless appendage. Very rarely, cancer of the lymph channels in the arm (lymphangiosarcoma) will result with dire consequences.

The patient's arm must be carefully protected after breast surgery. The shoulder must be exercised during the immediate post-operative period and the arm elevated on a pillow when sleeping.

One should not allow the arm to be used for taking blood samples or checking blood pressure, even after full recovery. Any minor injury to the fingers or hand should be attended to immediately. Sometimes oral medication to remove fluid and weight loss through diet control are helpful measures to control arm swelling.

Shoulder stiffness is due to inactivity because of pain and fear. If exercise is delayed, early scar tissue sets in after a few days, further restricting arm motion and ultimately leads to contractions. Often the doctor will arrange for the patient to visit a physical therapy clinic, where a therapist can outline a useful program. It's gratifying to note the patient's response and cooperation once she understands what is required.

With fewer radical mastectomies being performed in favor of the modified surgery, which leaves the large chest muscles intact, the shoulder stiffness is less of a problem. I also expect that fewer cases of severe arm edema (swelling) will be seen in the future since the modified surgery requires less dissection of the axilla.

Other complications to be aware of are caused by radiation. Depending on where the beam is directed one can sustain injury to nerves in the axilla (armpit)

Tamoxifen is finding a good deal of usefulness following the work of Dr Bernard Fisher and his colleagues.
• • • • • • •

leading to loss of function of the arm or hand. If radiation is directed to the chest wall there can be damage to the heart, lung, or ribs. Some patients have a persistent sore throat following radiation treatment that can last for weeks or months. Every effort is taken to prevent radiation complications and with newer techniques and better equipment these problems have been minimized. Severe nerve injury is largely a thing of the past, but radiation injury to the lung is still all too frequent.

PALLIATIVE TREATMENT OPTIONS

Palliative treatment is used in those cancer patients that can not be cured. The purpose of palliation is to relieve pain, bring comfort and extend life. For example in selected patients surgical removal of the ovaries followed by surgical removal of the adrenal glands or the hypophysis has been carried out with frequent lengthening of life. Chemotherapy and radiation are also used to control pain and extend life. These treatment methods must be weighed in the balance of benefit versus complications.

Surgery to remove the ovaries in my opinion is less hazardous than radiation because of possible radiation damage to the intestines and other organs with far reaching effects.

On the other hand, I would advise medical destruction of the adrenals since the surgical approach is beset with more potential complications.

Chemotherapy, used for both palliation and along with surgery to effect cure, can have significant complications such as loss of appetite, nausea and vomiting, and hair loss. The nausea usually subsides over time; and hair loss can often be prevented or delayed by the use of ice compresses and scalp tourniquet. By using a combination of chemotherapeutic drugs the dosage can be kept low and side effects avoided or minimized. The most serious complication of chemotherapy is bone marrow depression which can be irreversible.

The anti-estrogen, Tamoxifen is finding a good deal of usefulness following the work of Dr Bernard Fisher and his colleagues.[2] It is being used widely instead of removing ovaries, adrenals, or hypophysectomy in older women, and in younger women with certain criteria. Often standard chemotherapy is also employed at the same time.

PLASTIC SURGERY

Breast reconstruction following mastectomy means devising some method of reconstructing a mound to replace the breast tissue that had been removed. This could be accomplished by a pedicle of tissue brought forward from the back, or it may mean a free graft taken from the lower abdomen.

Although some surgeons pursue a course of immediate plastic repair at the time of initial breast amputation to lessen the psychological damage and avoid a later surgery, I would advise waiting at least six to eight months before a plastic procedure is attempted. This allows softening of scar tissue and full recovery from the cancer operation.

If plastic reconstruction is primarily undertaken to ease a sense of loss, there is a risk that the results can be less than optimal; and some women are even more distressed and fearful of facing family and spouse if the expectations of plastic surgery fall short. Therefore, it is important that a woman comprehend in

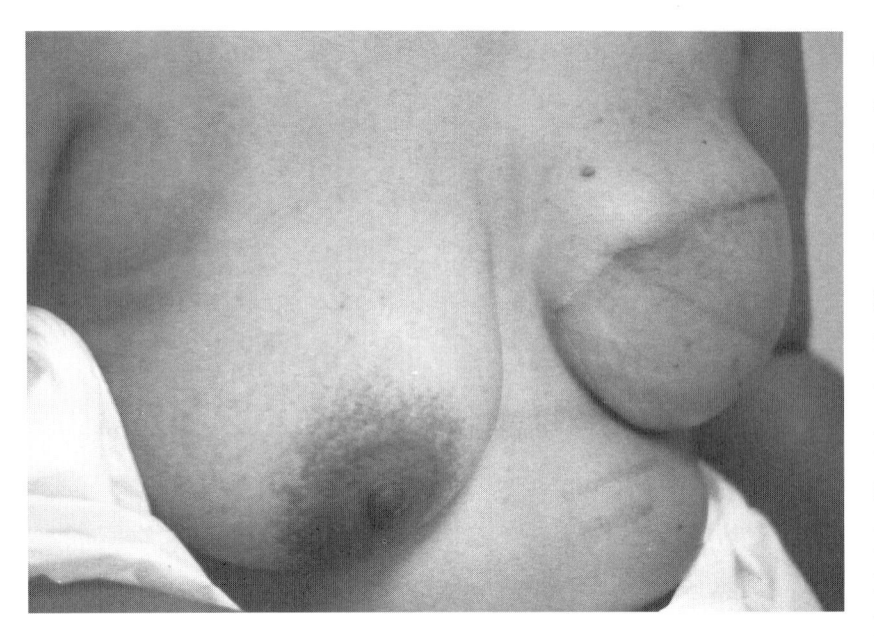

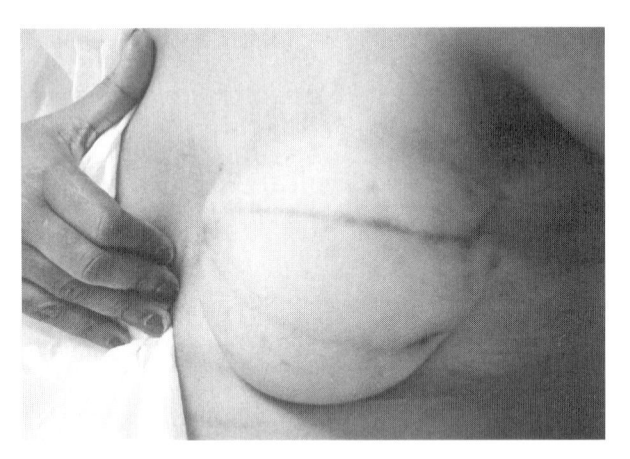

Fig. 8-2
Plastic Reconstruction of the Breast using the patient's own tissue. Muscle and fat can be shifted to the chest from the abdomen or flank and form an excellent breast mound that allows proper fitting of clothes as well as enhancing self-esteem in some patients.

detail all of the possible hazards and what the operation will and will not do. The patient must be given to understand in no uncertain terms that the purpose of plastic surgery is merely to provide a breast mound suitable to hold a comfortably fitted brassiere, to allow the proper fitting of clothes and to provide some semblance of balance and symmetry.

Insist that the plastic surgical procedure and results be illustrated with drawings, photos, and if possible by former patients. It would be helpful to talk to former patients who were happy with the outcome of plastic surgery as well as those women who were disappointed. If possible all sides of the issue should be examined. The prudent surgeon will avoid the "hard sell" or claim that plastic surgery can accomplish what it cannot. Remember, detectable wide spread metastasis or more than four axillary nodes positive for cancer argue against elective plastic surgery.

The plastic surgeon may elect to use muscle and skin flaps from the back, abdomen, or buttocks (Fig. 8-2 and Fig. 8-3). Or tissue expander techniques may be used. The decision is based on the circumstances of the particular case. Flap surgery should be thoroughly discussed to help the patient decide which approach would be appropriate.

In many cases breast reconstruction means the placing of a silicone filled plastic bag against the chest wall under the skin and scar or under the pectoral muscle (Fig. 8-4 and Fig. 8-5). However, experience in this area of plastic surgery has recently taken a serious back step as patients have come forth complaining of far-reaching complications.

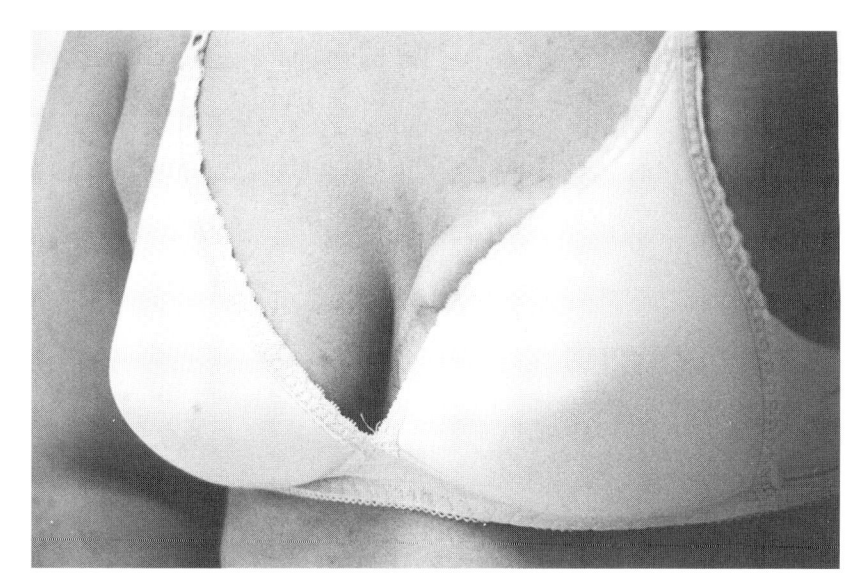

A frequent complication of silicone breast implantation is contracture and scarring. Of the 2 million women who have had silicone implants, capsular contracture rate as high as 74 percent has been reported, with obvious deformity and dissatisfaction.[3] In another series capsular contracture was found in 50 percent of cases. Dislocation of the silicone implant as well as leakage of the gel are also serious problems.[4]

In 1992, a temporary moratorium was levied against further use of silicone implants while investigation was being conducted to sort out the risks and complications.

Even when the oily silicone is replaced by saline there are not only the problems of the implant contracting and moving towards the axilla, there is also a deflation rate of 16 percent due to slow leakage.[5]

Let's examine some of the history of silicone im-

Fig. 8-3
Patient from 8-2 with bra in place. Tissue and muscle were shifted from the lower abdomen to the chest creating a suitable breast mound. At the same time unwanted fat was taken from the lower abdomen for a trimmer figure.

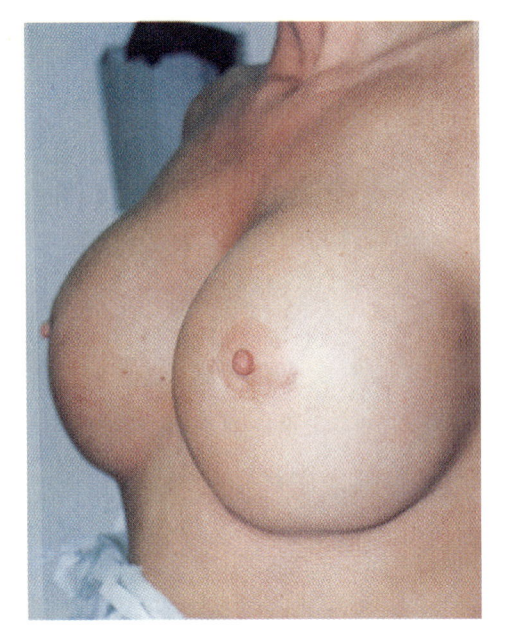

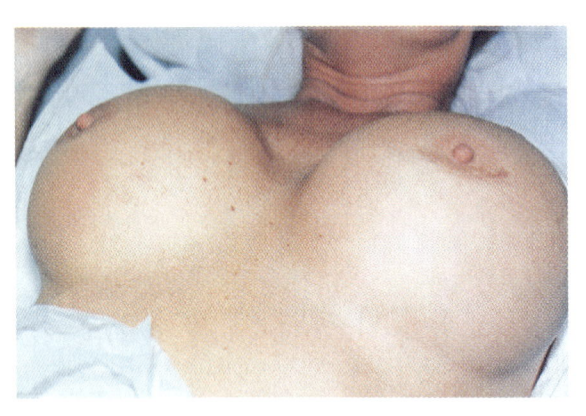

Fig. 8-4
Fifty year old patient with silicone placed under breast tissue for augmentation. This patient was operated a number of times because of the silicone implant drifting to the armpit or downward on the chest wall. These breast are very firm from the scar tissue that accumulates after surgery and even when reclining as in this photograph, the contour remains the same as when standing.

plants in this country. Before 1970, silicone, a synthetic oily clear liquid had been used to enlarge the female breast by direct injection. It found a market among entertainers and enjoyed a brief period of popularity. However, the free silicone in the tissue caused a severe reaction. Pain and inflammation occurred regularly. Abscess formation and draining ulcers were frequently reported. Before long, as you can imagine, the trend for silicone injection had run its course.

Then in the early 1970s silicone was sealed in plastic containers and placed under the breast tissue for breast augmentation. It was initially found to be quite acceptable with little side effect. From there it was only natural to suggest the use of contained silicone to reconstruct the breast after mastectomy. However, the operative principles had to be worked out. The guidelines for its application had to be written. Often the defect was enormous after radical mastectomy with the removal of such a large segment of tissue and muscle. So much skin was removed, that only a thin layer of tissue scarred to the ribs was left for the plastic surgeon. The medical profession had accepted the scar and tragic cosmetic results for seven generations in the attempt to cure cancer with radical surgery. Obviously the non-pliable skin and tissue following such surgery was not inclined to stretch over a plastic implant.

By 1975 Americans were becoming concerned and vocal about needless surgery and were asking for second opinions before submitting to a variety of proce-

154 LIGHTS, CAMERA, ACTION!

> *If you are considering silicone or a saline implant, remember that under the best of circumstances there are definite precautions to observe, and complications to anticipate. The pros and cons should be discussed early, even before mastectomy.*

dures, such as tonsillectomies and hysterectomies. It wasn't long before the need for radical mastectomy would be challenged. As mentioned in Chapter Seven, it was finally demonstrated that the modified radical mastectomy, removing less skin and tissue, and sparing the underlying muscles, had a comparable cure rate as the radical surgery.

With simple mastectomy and modified mastectomy becoming the preferred surgeries, it allowed for simpler plastic reconstruction. In fact by 1990 techniques were so improved that a growing number of patients were requesting reconstruction; and by that time most insurance carriers were providing coverage making breast reconstruction available for middle income patients as well as the poor.

As a matter of fact Maxine Waters (who has since become a Congresswoman) in California penned enabling legislation in 1980 that directed insurance carriers to cover reconstructive breast surgery following breast cancer surgery (AB 3548); and in 1984 Asemblywoman Waters introduced a bill directed at Medicaid (AB 2440) to provide the means to make this surgery also available to indigent patients.

In 1992 the roof caved in and further use of silicone implants was in jeopardy. As mentioned earlier a rash of serious complications were uncovered.

If you are considering silicone or a saline implant, remember that under the best of circumstances there are definite precautions to observe, and complications to anticipate. The pros and cons should be discussed early, even before mastectomy.

Immediate post-operative problems include bleeding into the operative site requiring drainage and perhaps re-operation. One must understand that infection, abscess and skin sloughing are all possible—

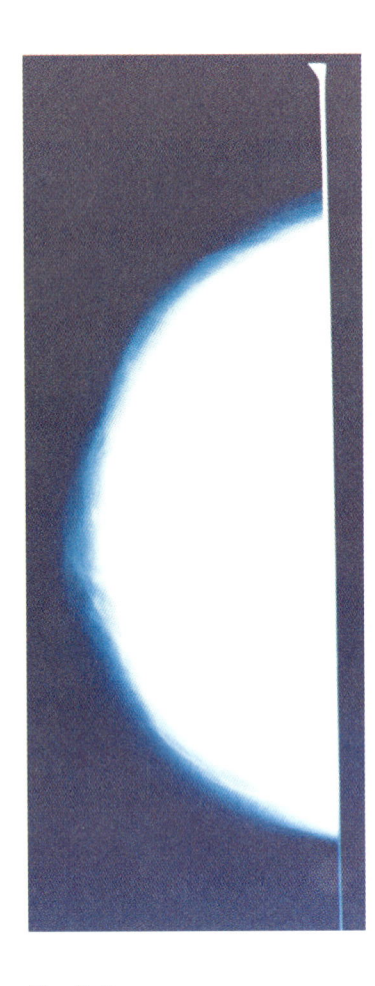

Fig. 8-5
Mammogram Showing Silicone Implant. Note the thin rim of breast tissue in front of the silicone. Detecting breast cancer in a breast that is distorted with silicone is very difficult and requires special techniques. Since a third or more of the breast can not be studied by mammography, careful and regular BSE is imperative.

even distortion and extrusion of the implant. There is still some controversy on how to handle the scar tissue forming around the implant which sometimes requires surgery to release fibrous bands. Anchoring the prosthesis to the chest wall can also be a problem. When done properly there is still a tendency for the implant to slide towards the axilla. Finally, the silicone may leak into the tissue causing irritation and inflammation.

The reconstructed areola-nipple complex derived from the labia adjacent to the vagina or from the opposite normal nipple does not carry its blood supply or nerve supply. In its new position the underlying blood vessels nourish it. The nerve supply does not rejuvenate and the graft is generally numb to the touch. If the normal breast was reduced in size to match the implant, the nipple may be transplanted upward to a new position to correspond to the position of the reconstructed nipple. Consequently, the normal nipple is also void of its nerve supply and is likewise numb to the touch. Or it may become infected and slough off completely.

The plastic surgeon must stress that it is impossible to match in configuration the opposite breast. No silicone implant can match a normal breast, The match can be enhanced by reducing the size and contour of the normal breast to approximate the contour of the silicone implant. There is also great difficulty in producing an areola-nipple complex to match the normal side. In some early cancers the nipple of the diseased breast was transplanted to another part of the body during mastectomy; and when breast reconstruction was carried out, the areola-nipple was placed in the appropriate location.

If the normal nipple-areola is large enough on the

Fig. 8-6
Patient is Wearing a Prosthesis in her brassiere following a right modified radical mastectomy. The prosthesis is a small spongy cushion that is roughly the same size as the opposite breast. It allows proper fitting and appearance of clothes.

normal breast, it may be partially excised and used to fashion a nipple for the reconstructed side. Others have used the skin near the vagina which may be dark, to make a suitable nipple for the reconstructed breast.

Plastic surgeons at the Medical College of Virginia report using dermabrasion exclusively in black women to darken the skin and placing a small piece of plastic under the center to simulate a nipple.[6]

Dermabrasion is simply the removal of the very top layer of skin which amounts to a superficial second degree burn. When it heals it leaves a darkened area. Then a small plastic chip is slid under the skin to the center of the darkened areola and an acceptable reconstructed nipple-areola is formed. This new procedure apparently is only applicable in black and other dark skinned women. Dermabrasion will not give a satisfactory darkening in fair-skinned women; but for black patients it is another tool available for the plastic surgeon.

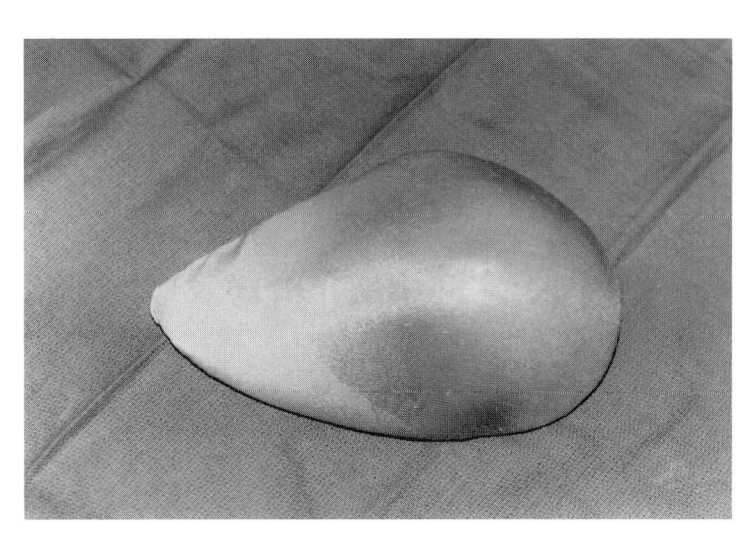

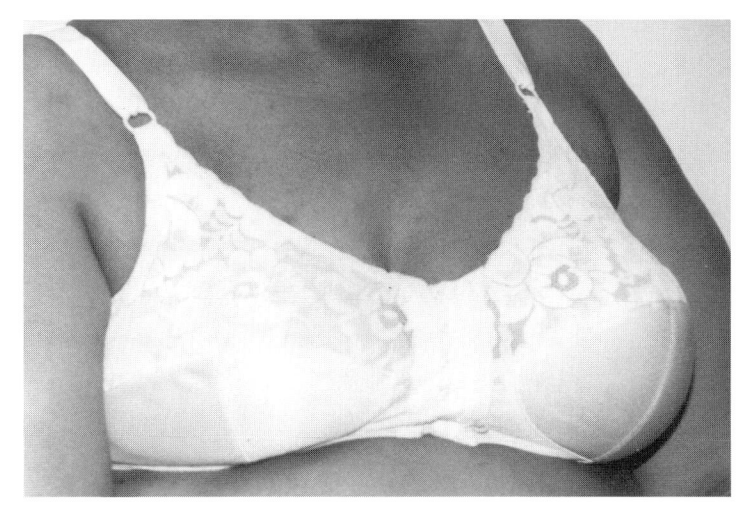

Many women, even under 40 years of age with an active sexual interest find a waning enthusiasm for plastic surgery as they adjust during the first few months after mastectomy. When the reconstruction procedure and possible complications are fully explained it is not uncommon for the husband and the patient to indicate their preference for postponement.

Most women will use a prosthesis worn in the brassiere. A variety of styles for all occasions have been developed and improved over the years. Various sizes and shapes are available in leading department stores across the country.

Nevertheless, some women desire reconstructive surgery or at least wish to know the possibilities available. Indeed these operations are getting better all the time and careful consideration with the plastic surgeon may be warranted. Be certain you understand what plastic surgery can and cannot do! Understand the risks and possible complications.

In coming years, I suspect, more women will be opting for lesser surgery, and preservation of the normal breast when the cancer is removed; and this will lessen the role of plastic surgery.

———

Along with concrete choices you must make about mastectomy, lumpectomy, plastic surgery, chemotherapy, radiation, Tamoxifen and other treatments, you must choose the right attitude and develop a positive point of view.

A personal physician can direct you to the right medical professionals that in turn will guide you through the first weeks of rehabilitation and decision making. That's fine. But you must come to grips with what is real in your life and what is nonsense. You must define what is important and what is simply a drag.

It's time to boldly step up on the stage of life, head held high. It's still your show, you know. Family and friends form a major part of the supporting cast of

Most women will use a prosthesis worn in the brassiere. A variety of styles for all occasions have been developed and improved over the years.

You must choose the right attitude and develop a positive point of view.
• • • • • • •

players. Only you can make it work.

After taking care of the tangible choices that lend themselves to a "Things to Do" list, you've got to get in to the realm of the psyche and the spirit. Actually it's the mystical side of your being that sustains you—that sustains all of us. It's what makes a singer like Abby Lincoln go on stage in spite of fever and physical weakness. Strength comes from the spirit and the will. No one quite understands it. It's a mysterious thing. Perhaps we get a bit closer to a definition when we marvel at the nature and handiwork of God that we witness all around us. Philosophers use parables and metaphors. Poets use rhyme and syntax. The preacher shouts from the pulpit; and we call on it through prayer and meditation. It is an invisible presence—impossible to describe. And yet it's that well that we must all tap to reap the fullness that life offers. I suppose it will always be mysterious. Like 'seeing through a glass darkly'. Some call it faith. 'The evidence of things not seen'. If you use it right it can sustain you and comfort you like a child knowing, 'Daddy won't let me fall'.

In the final analysis this life is **still** your show and the show must go on! It remains for you, only you, to take the time to remember and savor the good things and the blessings you've received in spite of adversity and pain. In spite of it all. It's still *you* who must find the inner strength and faith to go on. So study your lines and get ready for the rest of your life! Get up on that stage. Curtain's going up. Your audience awaits you. It's time for lights! It's time for camera! It's time for action!

REFERENCES

1. Fisher B Redmond C Brown A Wickerham DL Wolmark N Allegra J Escher G Lippman M Savlov E Wittliff J et al. Influence of tumor estrogen and progesterone receptor levels on the response to tamoxifen and chemotherapy in primary breast cancer. J Clin Oncol 1983 Apr;1(4):227-41

2. Gylbert L Asplund O Jurell G Capsular contracture after breast reconstruction with silicone-gel and saline-filled implants: a 6-year follow-up [see comments] Plast Reconstr Surg 1990 Mar; 85(3): 373-7

3. Plast Reconstr Surg 1991 May; 87(5): 879-84

4. Lemperle G Unfavorable results after breast reconstruction with silicone breast. Acta Chir Belg 1980 Mar-Apr; 79(2):159-60

5. Cohen IK: Reconstruction of the nipple-areola by dermabrasion in a black patient. Plastic Reconstruction Surg 67(2) Feb 1981 23-29

INDEX

A

Adrenal hormone (androstenedione)
Adrenalectomy / 116,129,131,132,150
Anatomy, breast / 23
    blood supply / 26,27
    glandular structure / 25,26
    lymphatic / 26,27
    muscles / 28
    veins / 26,27

B

Blood type and breast cancer
Breast development / 31
    in animals / 24
    in humans / 24
    milk glands / 24 milk ridges / 24,25
Breast self examination / 37-39

C

Cancers associated with breast cancer cancer in one breast / 66
    colon / 67
    leukemia / 67 ovary / 67
    salivary gland / 67
Cellular patterns of breast cancer and prognosis /104
    Combination / 106
    Ductal (infiltrating and in situ) /104
    Lobular (infiltrating and in situ) / 105
    Medullary /106
    Mucinous / 106
    Tubular /106
Chemotherapy / 128,131,147,150,151
    CAF (cyclophosphamide, Adriamycin, 5-florouracil) / 129
    CMF (cyclophosphamide, methyltrexate, 5-florouracil) /129
    L-pam (l-phenylalanine mustard) / 129
    Tamoxiphen / 131,151

D

Diagnosing Breast Cancer / 36,37,39
    biopsy / 148
    blood tests CEA / 54
    alkaline phosphatase / 53
    bone scan / 53
    chest x-ray / 53
    diaphanography / 50-51
    fibroadenoma / 42
    fibrocystic dysplasia 40
    mammography / 44-48
    nipple discharge / 51
    liver scan / 53
    thermography / 48
    ultrasound / 49-50
    DNA histogram / 54

E

Estrogen-receptor (ER) positive cancer / 129-132,135

Estrogen-receptor (ER) negative cancer / 129,132,135

F

Female hormones (ovary)
estradiol
estriol
estrone
FSH (follicle stimulating hormone) / 30,32
LH (leutenizing hormone) / 32
progesterone / 32

G

Guidelines for detecting breast cancer in asymptomatic women

H

Hormone control of breast / 29,30

Hormone therapy / 128

Hypophysectomy (surgical removal of the pituitary gland) / 131,132

I

Incidence / 59
of breast cancer in general / 59
of breast cancer in black women 59
of female lung cancer / 59 Immunotherapy / 132

L

Lobular carcinoma insitu / 65

M

Male breast cancer / 33
Menopause / 33
Menstrual cycle / 30
Mortality according to race / 59-60

P

Paget's Disease and Inflammatory Breast Cancer / 106,107

Plastic Surgery / 151,156,157
Breast prosthesis / 157
Breast reconstruction / 152
Silicone implants / 153-156

Progesterone-receptor (PR) positive cancer / 129,131

Prolactin / 70

R

Radiation alone / 125
complications / 127 with lumpectomy / 124-126

Reach to Recovery Program / 146

Rehabilitation / 147

Risk factors of breast cancer / 61
advancing age / 61
birth Control pills / 72
breast feeding / 63,64
female hormones produced in the body / 67
fibrocystic dysplasia / 65
diet / 74
gender / 62

heredity / 61
hormones for Hot Flashes / 71
injury / 63
parity / 63
racial genetics / 68,76-78
radiation / 64
socio-economic status / 78-81
smoking / 76
thyroid / 73

S

Screening populations for breast cancer / 88
    Breast Cancer Detection Demonstration Project (BCDDP) / 92,93
    Health Insurance Plan of Greater New York (HIP project) / 89
    Guttman Institute in New York (Dr Philip Strax) / 89-91

Staging Breast Cancer (TNM System) / 108

Surgery for breast cancer
    Radical Mastectomy (Halsted) / 115,117-121
    Partial mastectomy / 123
    Lumpectomy / 124 Modified radical Mastectomy / 121-123